◇◇◇◇◇◇◇◇◇◇◇◇◇◇◇◇◇◇◇◇◇◇◇◇◇◇〜〜〜〜

So You've Lost a Limb

By

D. A. Grady

◇◇◇◇◇◇◇◇◇◇◇◇◇◇◇◇◇◇◇◇◇◇◇◇◇◇◇◇◇

ISBN-13:978-1523350063
ISBN-10:1523350067

Cover Art by Angel Nichols
nicholsangel86@yahoo.com
http://www.angelwingsdesigner.com/bookcovers.htm

Disclaimer

So You've Lost a Limb is a nonfiction, heartfelt work, written by author and amputee D. A. Grady, based on his personal knowledge, lessons learned, and extensive coaching experiences. As such, the opinions expressed herein are those of the author and are intended only to benefit those facing the issues and concerns of an amputee's world.

Contents

The Story Begins

My name is D.A.Grady, and I'm an amputee.

For many of us, that statement is akin to the alcoholic introduction at every meeting of Alcoholics Anonymous. It's an acknowledgement, although somewhat different, that we're now able to tell the world that at least one of our body parts is no longer original equipment.

Many, if not most, amputees never grow completely comfortable with that admission, because it represents that we're somehow no longer equal to our peers and, in fact, are damaged goods, regardless of what wonders the medical world has done for us.

In the course of this book, I will try to shed light on the huge distance that develops, when a limb is lost, between an amputee and his or her loved ones and caregivers.

Please bear in mind that my amputation is a leg - below the knee (BK), so most of my references and experiences are in that arena. Subsequently, many of the examples I use focus on legs as my point of reference.

However, this book is written for all amputees, as the overall experience is similar for every person involved, when someone has lost a limb or body part in a way that is considered to be an amputation.

Before we get started, I want you to understand how broad a swath amputations cut in the very fiber of our country. In the United States, there are approximately 1.7 million people living with limb loss, either due to amputation or a congenital condition, and that number grows daily.

This book is my story, but it involves others, who now walk this path with me, amidst a growing number of folks who have lost or will lose a limb or limbs and those who will share their journey.

We amputees often share with others like us intimate thoughts and actions that we have learned to live with – the general ignorance of the public in dealing with us, as well as basic facts about how we go about living, including the disappointments and victories experienced, as we adapt and seek some level of comfort in our lives.

Mainly, this book is written to offer hope in the form of ideas, shared experiences, and practical suggestions for both sides of the equation to improve the total quality of life between all concerned - friends, family, caregivers and the amputee.

When a Limb is Lost

No matter when or how an amputation results, certain things occur beyond the patient's loss. Initially, due to heavy doses of medication, surgery and sleep, the amputee usually requires less attention than family, friends and loved ones.

Most hospitals deal quite poorly with taking the latter in tow and giving them a good basic training course on how to deal with their modified spouse, child or friend. According to most of these facilities, it isn't their job to fulfill this roll.

Instead, they point the newly born, involuntary caregivers towards various services, such as the prosthetic folks and other counseling agencies as future sources of information and to help them along the way. Consequently, those who must learn to deal with an amputee, wind up standing around the hospital room like bumps on a log.

Certainly, the prospective caregivers receive lots of love, spiritual-uplifting and well-wishing, along with sympathy.

Still, they don't get what they need because, as fast as facilities can, they slap a bandage on the new amputee, toss them into rehab, and send them home, often leaving them in the ill-equipped hands of the non-professionals who must now care for them, during the early stages of home recovery.

Suddenly, all those things done by a small army of trained hospital and rehab staff are thrust on the unsuspecting, uneducated caregiver, who may well be exhausted themselves from the supportive role they have been playing.

A mother, who bathed her young son years ago, now bathes that same child – a grown man who has lost his leg in a military operation.

A sister, who has never seen her grown brother naked, removes dirty underwear and washes her brother by hand.

An older husband, whose wife has always cared for him, is now forced into dealing with his wife's depression, about which he knows nothing, as the shock of her loss finally hits home with both him and her.

Many folks simply cannot handle these circumstances and others like them, creating a formidable wall that grows daily, until little is left of what had once been a strong relationship and neither party knows either why or what to do.

Certainly there are competent, professional caregivers for those in the small group who can afford them.

Generally speaking, the responsibility of caregiving falls on one or two members of the immediate family. It is an awesome task that, while it diminishes over time, never really goes away. Caregiving of amputees, in one form or another, is a lifetime mission!

Here's a snapshot.

Joe and Mary are in their late seventies and have been married for forty-five years. Joe has been an iron man all his life, made the money, and took care of pretty much everything.

Six months ago, he was diagnosed with sugar diabetes, and while the couple was getting acclimated to his medical routines, he fell, damaged his lower left leg, and it wouldn't heal.

Doctors informed the couple that his leg must be amputated below the knee. They went through the amputation process and learned what they could while he proceeded quickly through rehab. When the time came, neighbors took them home, since Mary had never learned to drive.

Once at home, Joe slid into a major depression, since he had never been sick a day in his life. On the other hand, Mary had never known a time when her iron man had not been able to take care of both of them, so she simply sat and waited for her Joe to recover and handle things again.

You can see how this goes. Joe never even tries to wear his new prosthetic device, even though he knows how to put it on. Mary doesn't know how to deal with the prosthetic, nor does she realize how depressed Joe is, and she doesn't understand why he isn't trying - a fact that scares her until she retreats even further away from him.

Friends and volunteers come by to help, but they have no idea where to begin, other than basic housekeeping and yard work, which both Joe and Mary object to, since they have always done those things themselves. So the visits slow down and eventually stop altogether.

With no input from the outside world, with the exception of some church folks bringing occasional dishes of food, they live on the few things that Mary buys from the store, when she can bum a ride with her neighbors.

Their life of many years begins to unravel, and they wind up spending the rest of their days as a married couple living separately in what was their home, missing out completely on what could have been golden years full of warmth, love and understanding.

Eventually, they die within a month of each other.

Fictional example? No. Unfortunately, this is a not so uncommon true story.

Getting Down to Nuts and Bolts

It is critical to understand a key part of most amputee's lives - the prosthetic.

As you continue to read, it will feel normal to refer back to this chapter, if for no other reason than to remind yourself of what an amputee goes through daily, at a minimum, to maintain a prosthetic limb.

In the flash of an accident or the decision of a doctor regarding a disease, a new function is introduced into a person's life. One might compare it to walking, which is relatively maintenance free, and then suddenly buying a car with all the attendant maintenance responsibilities that go with such ownership.

The newest prosthetic devices are marvels of medical and scientific engineering, but despite all that, they require basic care and maintenance that must be addressed daily for the remainder of an amputee's life. You heard it right - **daily for the rest of his or her life!**

No matter which limb has been amputated, there are certain pieces of equipment essential to the prosthetic. Generally, they are described like this in their order of use:

- *Liner* – exists to improve the amputee's safety and comfort by adding a cushioning layer between the residual limb and the prosthetic socket, more or less like a big sock.

- *Filler socks* – Various thicknesses, a kind of liner helper that's designed to take up any slack occurring between the liner and socket.
- *Socket* - The prosthetic socket joins your residual limb to the prosthesis and fulfills an important function. It ensures optimum adhesion to the liner and the proper fit of the prosthesis.
- *Prosthesis* - a device, either external or implanted, that substitutes for or supplements a missing or defective part of the body. It is connected to the bottom of the socket in various ways.
- *Sleeve* - holds the prosthesis firmly on the amputee, eliminating pistoning and/or bell-clapping as the leg swings during walking.
- *Footwear* – While we're in the neighborhood, what goes on the prosthetic foot needs some attention. You'll find that the artificial foot rarely is an even match for its natural counterpart, making the selection of shoes, boots, flip-flops or pretty much anything hard to match. Some folks even order two different sizes at some expense, just to get a good fit all around.

Guys like me hate to give up our cowboy type boots. In order to get them on and off, we have zippers installed, either on the side or back. I have found back zippers to be the best, simply because they don't get the same stress as those on the sides and, subsequently, last longer.

One final comment – It's important that you get a good solid fit so that maintaining balance is a normal part of your step and not something you have to labor with as you move about.

Here's a quick idea of what I and other amputees face daily.

Occasionally, the liners become slippery with perspiration, depending on physical exertion. Because muscles expand with exertion and then shrink when at rest, we may have to add or remove a layer of filler socks at various times throughout the day.

Sleeves may develop a wrinkle or bubble that must be smoothed out and pulled tight again to ensure a snug fit, so that the prosthesis won't become loose or fall off. (Had that happen to me once while mowing the grass. Hopped back to it, sat down, put it on, and prayed that no one had seen me. When my wife got through laughing, she told me she had. It was funny, even to me.)

Most of these cases involve complete removal of the prosthesis. Unless the amputee carries extra socks and a hand towel to dry his or her prosthetic limb and stump, they won't be able to deal with such situations independently and appropriately.

Are you beginning to get a small inkling of what amputees face, day and night?

One more thing. Generally, we can do almost anything we could've done pre-amputation, but not without constantly reminding ourselves that we must be very deliberate in everything that we do.

My rule is: ***Think through it, before you do it.*** Works every time.

Snapshot – One

- Generally speaking, the responsibility of caregiving falls on one or two members of the immediate family.
- Caregiving of amputees, in one form or another, is a lifetime mission!
- It is critical to understand a key part of most amputee's lives - the prosthetic.
- The newest prosthetic devices are marvels of medical and scientific engineering, but despite all that, they require basic care and maintenance that must be addressed daily for the remainder of an amputee's life. You heard it right - **daily for the rest of his or her life!**
- Liners can become slippery with perspiration, depending on physical exertion.
- Unless the amputee carries extra socks and a hand towel to dry his or her prosthetic limb and stump, they won't be able to deal with such situations independently and appropriately.
- Think through it, before you do it. Works every time.

Chapters for the Ages

These next few chapters are designed to take you through the lives of amputees at various ages.

Each group will reflect remarkable differences in the impact such a loss has on their lives. The lessons contained for you as potential caregivers, loved ones, or friends will be painfully clear and will tug at your heartstrings, I promise.

No one is immune from becoming an amputee.

File that statement away.

By the way, are you aware of the fact that removal of a breast and subsequent implants for mental health sake fall into the amputee category? Kind of changes the playing field, doesn't it?

The same issues confront these patients as with any other amputee, except they have issues unique to themselves. We'll talk about that some on down the road.

In the pages that follow, I will show you both sides of the amputee equation:

- **Amputees (AMs)** – How they confront the fact that a removal of one of their crucial parts is required and how they live with it, and

- **Caregivers(CGs), family members, friends, and fellow workers** - How little they know what they will be asked to do and give, in order for the amputee to mentally and physically adapt to living life in ways never before dreamed of by either side.

Both of the above are faced with life-long commitments that they never imagined. In their pasts, they often had come face-to-face with what we, as a society, call the handicapped, gave them a brief moment of pity, thanked the powers that be they were not among them, and then moved on with their lives.

There are those infrequent moments when we must explain to our young children what has happened to a handicapped person we just passed on the street or watched as they struggled to climb a flight of stairs.

"Now, don't stare at people like that, honey," we say. "The poor person has lost an arm or leg due to some unfortunate mishap, and we must feel compassion or even pity for them."

And so, the conversation ends.

Why not pass out a little praise and admiration for the person, whose life has been unalterably changed?

"Now, don't stare like that, honey. Just think what a wonderful person he or she must be. Living with a missing limb must be really hard."

Just saying...

On Being a Child Amputee

This chapter's title is kind of easy to say, but much harder for the child involved to come to grips with.

From the time anyone, child or adult, loses a limb for whatever reason, their understanding really boils down to varying shades of how the situation they now face developed.

Let's start with a child, who has been born with a limb deformity.

Over time, despite probable harassment by their peers, he or she will become accustomed to their condition and learn to live with it in a comfort zone of sorts that works for them. They will have learned and now understand their limitations, and each of them will have worked out their own formula for making it through life.

Enter Mom, Dad and medical science, all striving to improve the child's condition.

Many parents have a much harder time dealing with their child's infirmities than the child does. If an opportunity arises to improve their child's well-being, including replacing the deformity with a prosthetic, some parents will jump at it, with little thought or knowledge as to what the child thinks or desires.

Sadly, there are even parents who approach such possibilities as a way to improve the look of their family.

Whatever their motivation, parents are often totally unprepared for the transformation in their child.

No matter the type of amputation - be it cosmetic, due to disease or an accident of some sort - the child will have two basic concerns:

1. How much will it hurt?
2. How will people, mainly their peers, react to it?

The child should be told up front that, yes, it will hurt a lot, but only for a short period of time. Most youngsters live in the now, which equates to a short period of time for them, so the pill they are being requested to swallow becomes less bitter through this approach.

The second is harder. Children tend to live in a world of their own equality, meaning they should look and act like everybody else their age, so their acceptance is guaranteed.

The sole exception to that scenario is race. From their inception, children are color blind. They do not see black, red, yellow, tan or any other color as a qualification for equality. Another reason why it comes as such a shock to them that their classmates are suddenly not equal, once they have experienced an amputation.

Adults teach them that color impacts equality in their lives, whether we mean to or not. I believe, as do many others, that human nature makes us fear what we do not understand, and studies are showing that this is the very basis of prejudice.

Children's sensory factors are maxed out from birth. After all, they have a lot of catching up to do to fit into today's world.

Words are not the only things that influence a child. Sighs, askew glances, withdrawal, avoidance and many other actions from adults, all signal acceptance or denial of any specific reference to equality, and there are many others - all sensed and dealt with in a child's brain at an amazing speed.

Another major factor for acceptance in a child's world of look-alike is the two arms, two legs, and one head (TATLOH) syndrome. I made that up, but it works.

Suddenly, a child wearing a prosthetic shows up in class. Even with a proper introduction by the teacher, a new student or even more important, a former classmate and friend is suddenly different to the other children.

For argument's sake, let's say the new kid in class is not new, just different, because now he or she has a strange device attached to them. That person no longer qualifies by the TATLOW manifesto. In case you are wondering, the disfigured limb we just talked about, qualified, because the child was born with it.

As is the very nature of children, who have been unconsciously taught by their parents, now this former friend no longer qualifies as being equal, and taunting, bullying, teasing and general shunning of the new amputee often begins.

"What's the matter, Johnnie, can't you run?"

"Betsy, you're a gimp."

And so, it goes - cruelty to the max, but not something the other children can control, because of their upbringing and fear of the unknown.

The child amputee now wears a yoke from which many of them will never be free, only one of the issues facing a child amputee.

Here's another example and some good advice. It is important because of its difference from the above. How about the amputee child who doesn't want a prosthetic?

I recently became aware of this situation, and information relayed to me by the father of this wonderfully impressive young lady, bears repeating. Their doctor told them that some children take to a prosthetic and some don't.

The young lady in question didn't want one then, and even after she expressed some interest in one during her middle school years, she felt it was too much bother and to this day doesn't wear one. Her amputation was done as a baby, removing her right arm below the elbow.

It wasn't easy for her. As a young child, even before and certainly through elementary and middle school, she would withdraw whenever anyone asked her about her missing limb. Her parents sat down and wrote a very simple, but ingenious *I was sick and this resulted* statement that was easy for his daughter, even as a small child, to remember.

Knowing that all she had to do was repeat this statement, gave her the confidence to stand up and do so, and other children readily accepted it as a sufficient response from her, their curiosity satisfied. Also, her new found confidence helped to keep her from being bullied because she was different.

Since children adapt to such things in general easier than adults, they reported she never missed having a right hand – in the same way that being born blind is different from going from being sighted to being blind.

I had a hard time with that one.

Fierce independence from assistance in areas beyond the amputation is quite normal as the child works through the path that is emerging for them. As a cautionary note, I suggest letting them go until they ask for help and not forcing it on them, just as with any amputee.

They also said that the child would occasionally hit out at others with her stump. Maybe it was a way of self-expression, but such actions must be handled with the same love and discipline you would administer to any child misbehaving. Singling them out will do more harm than good.

This young person is now a junior in high school and shopping for a college. It appears to me that this family healed themselves together, finding the best for their daughter and quite possibly the best for themselves as well.

It is a wonderful example of how to make amputations work out successfully.

Many lose their way along the path to adulthood, simply because the role models they had depended on no longer fill or are capable of filling that need. They have never been confronted with their child's problem. Parents can and should learn everything possible about the new issues they face as a family, but many do not. Whatever their reason, it's a pitiful excuse.

When their parents can no long respond to a child's need to learn, grow, and adapt, those children flounder and often fail at the task of living, through no fault of their own. In truth, no one individual is at fault, as the situation is the direct result of a society that has failed to shepherd every sheep in the flock, not just the general majority.

For a child desperately seeking equality in life, this is a slippery slope that often deprives society of brilliant minds and talents, forcing a promising child into a life of mediocrity and, in some cases, massive depression and an early death.

Amputations Resulting from Wounds

Before you lose all hope, let me show you some good news. Wounded Warriors, while suffering the hideous results of war, have once again carried the banner for our country and many others. The sheer volume of their amputations has caused a major increase in the type and quality of medical and technical help that is now available to all.

A wise man once said, "It takes a war to awaken the medical community to the needs of all those who suffer."

Never has that been more true than today. Travel with me for a moment to the Olympics and countless other television and media presentations, where amputees have proven time and time again that they can not only compete, but excel, in many areas of life never dreamed of before.

The medical community has shifted gears. New products provide increased functionality to nearly anyone in the form of hands, arms, legs, feet, breasts, and even implants of the eye itself.

For the first time, the amputee community is beginning to feel empowered, as it comes closer and closer to equality with its peers, leveling the playing field for all.

This poor pen cannot adequately define such an impact on the world's population. Our childhood amputees see these young dynamos competing on the athletic field, as well as in the workplace, and become fired with their own potentials, possibly for the first time in their lives.

Excitedly, they seek parental counsel as to how they, too, can look, act and be as accomplished and successful as the fine examples they have now witnessed.

Unfortunately, there is a brick wall.

Previously, I said available to all, and that is true. Unfortunately, available is not the same as accessible or even advisable for this or that individual.

There are horrendous voids of information that deny people of all ages access to such assistance. The spider web of missing or confusing facts about getting help, turns many away. Then, too, there is the sheer mountain of costs, unclimbable by many.

Have things improved in recent years?

Yes, but in this, the greatest country in the history of mankind, we have barely begun to address the issue of putting all amputees on a level playing field with the rest of us.

Are we seeing a significant growth of mechanically aided people in the workforce? Absolutely.

We are headed in the right direction, but there is an entire generation of vital young people who could and would make ours a better nation, who are still being denied their chance.

As a result, there are increasing numbers of young Americans, who are retreating into their old world of non-equality and mediocrity - a loss not only to them, but to the rest of us. In some ways, they make up the home of the brave more than most, simply because of the battles they fight daily to survive in our world.

Imagine the bravery it must take to face every day knowing that your life could be lived normally, but not knowing how to get there. We'll look long and hard at this conundrum in chapters to come.

In the meantime, let's explore the world of older Americans, our seniors, who also face the world of amputeeism with a completely different set of rules by which they now must play.

Amputation by Illness

Until recently, when large numbers of wounded warriors with amputations began returning home, the largest group affected by amputation were those suffering from sugar diabetes, although there are other diseases that can result in one or more amputations as they progress.

It has been my experience that most of these folks are senior citizens, and their situations are compounded by their ages, the underlying disease itself, and figuring out how to deal with the many aspects of this new burden on their already bent shoulders.

Stop and consider this a moment.

Here you are, in your sixties or older, already having to deal with the aches and pains of getting older. Some doctor has told you that you have diabetes, and you now must take insulin or some other medication. The very thought of sticking yourself with a needle turns your stomach.

As you try hard to get into the routine required of you, there is a slight accident which leaves some cuts and bruises on your foot. Previously, this would have been a short term concern, but now your minor injuries don't seem to heal.

For medical reasons that you don't completely understand, the doctor tells you that he will have to **remove your big toe**.

At home, after a big jolt of whiskey, you convince yourself that it won't be such a big deal, since you have nine other toes to depend on. You agree, and the surgery is done.

You betcha folks, this is an amputation, and in many more cases than I care to remember, it is the first of several.

I generally meet such folks after they have already had several operations, and the next one will mean taking the leg at the knee or higher.

How do I meet them? Let me explain.

After I lost my left leg below the knee (BK) back in 2006, I felt very obligated to the young surgeons who were willing to save the rest of my leg, because it had been in pretty tough shape, too.

I was mighty lucky to have a quick (relative term) recovery, and I suspect these young doctors knew I would help out if I could, because they approached me with a question. In response, I gladly agreed to counsel other amputees if it would help.

Little did I know in the beginning, that counseling them would help me far more than those with whom I spoke.

Bottom line: That is how I wind up in the homes or at hospital bedsides of so many folks in post amputation circumstances.

The senior amputee is confronted with an entirely different set of circumstances than anyone else. Most of them are receiving Medicare, which covers many of the expenses of the surgical procedures and limited in-home assistance. In addition, Medicare supplement policies as well as drug RX programs help to offset costs.

For anything beyond that, a senior citizen is pretty much on his or her own.

Those unfortunates, whose required services aren't covered by Medicare or who are unable to afford supplemental insurance, face an almost insurmountable cost. Generally, they can do little or nothing to help themselves, as they are already living on a fixed income.

If they do get some kind of assistance, it often is in a facility that provides subpar care and treatment.

During the productive parts of their lives, these folks held regular jobs, raised families, and chased the American dream like the rest of us. Looking towards their Golden Years, they had figured that, with Social Security, maybe a retirement pension, and a part time job, they could survive.

Additionally, we now have an ever-growing group of mature citizens, who have lost good jobs as a result of our current economy and, simply because they are over fifty, have been unable to find a new position.

None of us ever figures an amputation into the equation of living, and subsequently, we make no effort to find out anything about it, barring the tales we hear. When the day comes to make a decision for amputation or face the new reality of one we didn't expect, near panic sets in.

In my case, the amputation was performed without my permission when I hit and removed a section of guard rails. When it was over, I remember vividly seeing my cowboy boot, leg still in it, sitting on the dash of my truck. My first thought was "Well, I'll be damned."

The good news?

I didn't have to make the decision about whether I wanted my left leg removed below the knee or not. Right from the jump, I was one step ahead of most, as there would be no recriminations later about my having made a wrong decision.

I get occasional calls from doctors or prosthetists asking me to stop by and visit a recent amputee. Walk with me as I meet one of them in his home. This particular gent had lost both legs below the knee and met me at the door in his wheelchair.

When I make such visits, I usually wear a pair of cowboy boots and jeans. With a bit of concentration, I walk with little, if any, limp. So it was on this day.

I introduced myself to the gentleman, who told me his surgeon had told him I would be coming.

As we got settled, I explained to him I had been asked to visit with him about his amputations. His question was the same as every other person I counsel.

"What do you know about amputations?" he asked.

My reply was to pull up my pant leg and show him my prosthesis.

His eyes widened. "I would never have known. How did you learn to walk so well?"

My answer was direct. "First, I had to get out of bed and off my wheelchair, and the rest came by itself, with a lot of work."

"I don't have either leg."

Noticing two new-looking prosthetics in a corner, I asked for permission to examine them. There wasn't a mark on either. "Have you ever tried them on?"

"Not by myself. The therapy folks showed me some things at the hospital and then kinda disappeared after I got home."

"Well, I'm here," I pointed out. "Will that do?"

Over the course of the next hour, we got both his prosthetic legs on, and I helped him to his feet. When I asked how they felt, there were tears in his eyes.

"They hurt some, but in a good way."

I knew exactly how he felt, and with him holding my arms and me walking backwards, he took his first few steps in his own home.

I went back several more times to teach him about taking care of his 'new' legs. He started by using a walker for additional support and balance control, then two canes and, finally, nothing.

I can't tell you which of us felt better about his change of circumstances.

On my last visit in the series, he met me at the door wearing his prosthetics, proud as a peacock, a wonderful smile on his face. It was my turn for tears.

Over the years, I've gone back several times, just to check on him.

Now bathing himself and maintaining his prosthetics correctly, he has a housekeeper, and meals-on-wheels comes regularly. He takes a handicapped bus to do his own shopping. Most impressive to me is that he has re-engaged with life. Go, Mr. G!

His is now a life he can live with and, you can tell from the smile on his face, that he has reached a point of relative happiness.

As for me, I'm so proud of him and, frankly, of me, too. It sure feels good.

Such situations don't always turn out that well, because there aren't enough people, including family members, who will show up at the door of an amputee and say, "Let's get you walking."

The focus of this book is AMs, CGs and their attendant families. Obviously, there's a segment of the AM world where an AM, who lives alone, comes out of the hospital and goes home wherever that may be.

It is crucial for you to reach out immediately for help and support!

Even with a strong support group, life is difficult for a new AM. *Without that help, nearly impossible.*

Here are a few places where support can be found and, perhaps, help you to develop a network of people who can and will assist you:

- The case worker assigned to you by the hospital.
- Other AMs and their families you might meet while in the hospital.

- The prosthetists assigned to help you get a new prosthetic.
- Churches and civic clubs you may belong to or know of.
- Groups made up exclusively of AMs – and there are many who can be found through your prosthetics agency.

From your contacts with these folks, there is usually a path that develops to guide you towards the CG community and the type of support every AM requires.

Amputation by Accident

As we start this section, I want to tell you another of my experiences. I got a phone call from one of the surgeons who had worked on my leg, asking if I would visit a young man who had lost a leg as a result of a motorcycle accident.

This man was still in the hospital when I went calling. As I walked into his room, he was arguing with an unfeeling bill collector who had called.

Now this young fellow had no support group of any kind, and between the trauma of his accident and all the issues of dealing with his insurance or lack thereof, he was extremely angry, as I would have been in the same situation.

I sat by the door until he shouted at the phone and hung up.

Looking at me, he growled, "Now, what do you want?"

I explained why I was there at his doctor's request, and he responded, (same verse, later chapter) "What the hell do you know about it, if you ain't no doctor?"

I pulled out my ace and eased my pant leg up a bit.

He said nothing for a minute, then asked, "How can you walk like you do with that thing on?"

Using my stock answer, I believed I had impressed him, but his anger remained. He didn't give a damn about anything.

"Can I see your stump?" I stepped forward.

"No."

"I just wanted to see if yours was any uglier than mine."
He kinda smiled.

This was a big, old, healthy country boy, who was just a little nervous about some old guy wanting to look at his leg.

To ease the tension, I told him, "I'll bet a ten dollar bill that mine's uglier than yours."

That did it.

He slid that stump out from under the sheet, and it was beautiful, as amputations go.

You see, surgeons can do all kinds of things to pretty up a stump. When you lose a leg as I did, it's just plain uglier than yesterday's lunch, and there isn't much anyone can do about it.

I looked at him. "I'm gonna be sorry to take your money." I dropped my trousers and slid my prosthetic off.

"Damn, Mr., that's the ugliest thing I've ever seen."
We both laughed.

Getting dressed, I walked him through the process of putting his prosthesis on right and asked if he had worn his yet.

He shook his head, and after some cajoling, I got him into it.

I could tell that it was a little painful, but he never said a word, as he tested his weight on it and then took a couple of steps along the wall.

Long story short, by the time I left, he had walked half the length of the hospital corridor and back.

He was tired, but there was a smile on his face.

"I'll be back tomorrow." I stood to go.

"It's okay, Mr. I got this."

He hadn't said thanks, but none was required.

I never saw him again, but I did get a call from his surgeon a few days later, asking me what I had told him. Laughing when I asked why, the doctor said the man had checked himself out the morning after my visit and left the hospital.

I did find out later that this guy had signed into a rehab center and was doing fine.

Attempts to help a recent amputee in the same mental state as this fellow was don't always turn out as well as this one initially did, so you enjoy the ones you can and move on.

Some folks have no support group of any kind. It makes no difference how old or young an amputee is, if they don't have someone to share their situation, most simply shrivel up and lose hope. They become recluses and, quite often, die alone and in pain.

That is the saddest of all situations. No human being should have to live his or her life alone, grieving, bewildered, and afraid!

Let me remind you what an amputee deals with every day – often multiple times a day.

We talked earlier about the working parts of most prosthetics and what it takes to keep them in working order – no small feat.

Starting with getting up in the morning, there are several steps that must be done, every time you remove or put on a prosthetic.

First, comes the inspection of the stump where the amputation occurred.

An amputee must look for any signs of abrasion, calluses, blisters or open sores. If some exist, they must be treated from a never-ending chest of medical supplies. If you have limited movement in your stump, this step may require a mirror.

This can pose its own problems, for you have taken your leg off to go to bed, so all medications must be kept in or near your bed stand, and that includes handy wipe type towels for scrubbing the stump.

Author's note: I heartily suggest that you go to the bathroom before going to bed.

When I first was learning about such things, I was awakened early one morning with an urgent need to empty my bladder.

Without a moment's hesitation, I rolled sleepily out of bed, took one step, and realized too late that there was nothing there with which to take a second one. I kind of slid down the wall like a wet pickle, trying desperately to keep from wetting all over everything and then valiantly crawled to the toilet.

Lesson learned – Always go to the bathroom one last time before bed. It's also a good idea to practice putting your leg on fast for possible future events – your wife hearing a burglar downstairs or a fire.

I've got it down to three seconds – not always right, but workable, and I haven't had any further issues on that subject.

Putting on the leg in all its glory:

First thing that goes on most any amputated limb is the liner. This necessity needs to have been cleaned thoroughly. Roll it up on your stump, making sure that there are no bubbles or wrinkles.

Then slide the prosthetic socket on, just to test and make sure the fit is snug. If it isn't snug, remove the thing and add layers of socks, testing each sock with the socket until it fits properly.

Finally, roll the sleeve up over the socket, until it reaches a point on your limb where it can hold the entire prosthetic in place and not let it slide down.

Now that you have seen how that works, let's take into account that sweat, exertion and a multitude of other factors can cause the sleeve and socket to loosen. Be prepared to adjust the prosthetic multiple times each day, going through the general above process each time.

Are you getting the picture?

And yet, we amputees are willing to put ourselves through this repeated regimen, because nearly all of us wish to stay in the game of life with the rest of you, even though our choices are limited, as you have read.

I have used a leg prosthetic for these examples as that is my expertise. I know that other limbs have their own peculiarities – some worse, some better than my situation. Just wanted you to be aware of that as well.

One final note on an amputee's daily life. **He or she can never take that synthetic limb for granted.** It must always be foremost in our minds, as a conscious part of the deliberate approach to life that we now must take.

Can we dance, run, hunt, fish, ride horses, drive cars, climb ladders, or the myriad of other things that non-amputees do? You can bet your booties on it! Just a little more deliberately, that's all.

Still, these pleasures and more, must be done with an amputee's thought processes always asking the question, "How will my next move affect or be affected by my prosthesis?"

Snapshot – Two

- Why not pass out a little praise and admiration for the person, whose life has been unalterably changed?
- Many parents have a much harder time dealing with their child's infirmities than the child does.
- No matter the type of amputation - be it cosmetic, due to disease or an accident of some sort - the child will have two basic concerns:
  1. How much will it hurt?
  2. How will people, mainly their peers, react to it?
- The child should be told up front that, yes, it will hurt a lot, but only for a short period of time.
- The child amputee now wears a yoke from which many of them will never be free, only one of the issues facing a child amputee.
- Some children take to a prosthetic and some don't.
- Sit down and write a simple, explanatory statement that's easy for the child amputee to remember.
- There are increasing numbers of young Americans, who are retreating into their old world of non-

equality and mediocrity - a loss not only to them, but to the rest of us.

- The senior amputee is confronted with an entirely different set of circumstances than anyone else.
- It is crucial for an AM, who lives alone, to reach out immediately for help and support!
- It makes no difference how old or young an amputee is, if they don't have someone to share their situation, most simply shrivel up and lose hope. They become recluses and, quite often, die alone and in pain.
- Starting with getting up in the morning, there are several steps that must be done, every time you remove or put on a prosthetic.
- First, comes the inspection of the stump where the amputation occurred.
- It's also a good idea to practice putting your leg on fast for possible future events – your wife hearing a burglar downstairs or a fire.
- An AM can never take that synthetic limb for granted. It must always be foremost in our minds, as a conscious part of the deliberate approach to life that we now must take.

Caregiving vs Care-Taking

Caregiving is not taking care of someone. That is care-taking. Taking care of someone implies doing work on or for a person in an impersonal, clinical way, without deep affection or one-on-one caring. It is purely what the name implies.

It is the kind of care you receive in a hospital or rehab center, where you are simply another of the many patients that person has been assigned to on any given day. They have read your chart and perhaps chatted with your doctor about your case.

They bring you shots and pills, help you get in and out of bed when you are ready, and then assist you with your ablutions.

In a couple of days, they introduce you to your therapist, whose job it is to teach you about prosthetics in general. These folks do preliminary measuring and chat with the medical staff.

Such persons are also care-takers. If you don't think so, find a recent amputee who's still in the hospital, locate their nurse or therapist, and ask them how much they know about their patient. Their answers will confirm what I'm saying.

To recap, a new amputee in a hospital has met and been taken care of by doctors, nurses, aides, attendants and therapists at a minimum, most or none of whom know anything at all about caregiving for the person. It is simply not a part of what they are trained to do.

Unfortunately, a vast number of people fall into the category of being a care-taker, not a caregiver, and the difference between the two is night and day. As I said, taking care of someone is almost clinical in nature, and most of the medical people I have dealt with, took great care of me and others I have known, but did not give care.

A caregiver does so much more than taking care of someone. Whether short or long term, a true caregiver becomes a part of that person's life in every detail, from the physical things that must be attended to, through the emotional highs and lows, that person travels each and every day.

Caregivers get to know all about you and familiarize themselves with the key people in your life. Often they make contact with your support group to help and explain exactly what it is they are doing for you.

To give you a perfect example of caregiving, my mother-in-law lived with us in the last period of her life. We were extremely fortunate in finding two women who were the epitome of caregiving. When family members showed up to visit, they met them, learned about them, and kept contact with them.

They asked my wife and I endless questions about mother's past, her likes and dislikes, and then taught us about what they were doing and how to do it ourselves. If one of us became ill, they showed up and pulled extra shifts to make certain Mom received constant care.

You could see the affection they felt for all of us, particularly Mom, who would light up when either of them entered her room. Truly, there was love all around.

When Mom passed, it was only minutes before both of them showed up to bath and prepare her body. As a testimonial to their caring, there was not a single bed sore on her body, because during those final days, they had turned and moved her every couple of hours.

They remain in our lives to this day.

That is Care-Giving!

Amputee Caregiving

What follows will be my attempt at clarifying caregiving for an amputee. It differs somewhat from the example I have just given.

A crucial piece of the process, caregiving must be known and applied in each instance of an amputee's life. Although such care is not limited to folks like the ones I mentioned above, it should specifically include family members such as spouses, children, close relatives and friends. Each of them must become caregivers of sorts in order for the new situation to work.

While not all forms of caregiving deal with the physical tasks of helping an amputee, they do require in-depth knowledge of that person's physical and mental state. Amputees rarely require round-the-clock attention and often need little, if any, daily assistance, once they have come to terms with their situation.

However, during the primary adjustment from hospital to home and beyond, some forms of professional help are normally required. During such times, a hired caregiver can provide service to the amputee as well as equally important education to spouses and other family members. The best professionals teach all involved in the new situation by example and through discussions.

Fulfilling their primary goal, these persons will teach the basic skills required of the amputee, before he or she can return to some kind of normalcy in their lives.

At the same time, they can train those who will become the amputee's support system in the skills necessary for them to provide similar caregiving long term, once the professionals are gone. In many cases, because of differences among family members and/or friends, this expanded training can be more difficult to achieve than working with the patient.

Dealing with the entire support group of an amputee often means being in a place where different emotional roller-coaster rides are going on simultaneously for each member present. Most differences are driven by ignorance, but many are anger or fear oriented, because of the unknowns an amputee brings home with them. These potential caregivers truly love the amputee, but…

While training extended support persons to deal with the physical issues of a prosthesis, caregivers must find and deal with the issues confronting each member. If issues remain, the chances of the amputee, as well as their family and friends, regaining any kind of normalcy for living are greatly diminished.

Let me give you some examples.

Let's start with the spouse, since they are the ones who usually bear the brunt of the load in any family.

Without love, the entire situation becomes much more difficult. Two people who love each other and have learned to share their lives together are way ahead of the game.

Such couples seem to mind meld and send signals to one another, letting each know the other is there for them no matter what. I cannot emphasize the importance of that statement enough.

These lucky couples seem to think together, when dealing with all phases of their new circumstances. Each lets the other know that, regardless of what has happened, they will make it – together. A beautiful thing to see happen, unfortunately it is not viewed often enough.

Children or parents of an amputee have a higher hill to climb, because of a couple of words – pity and fear.

Pity is the worst enemy of an amputee.

Pity compounds existing issues and can deny the amputee the ability to return to as close to a normal lifestyle as possible.

Amputees get very angry when shown pity. The pitier fails to understand why and gets angry in turn. Thus a vicious circle is begun.

It makes little difference to an amputee who is doing the pitying. Anger is involuntary on their part, because it is usually translated into blame for the situation.

Therefore, the first lesson to be learned in the care and feeding of an amputee is eliminate pity or in the vernacular of today: **No more pity parties.**

The best way to accomplish this goal is to let the amputee explore his or her limits.

This exposure to pity happened to me after I lost my leg. My children hired a lawn service for my house out of concern for my safety. It upset me greatly, because managing my yard had always been therapeutic for me.

When I mentioned it to my wife, she was consoling, saying that the kids were only concerned for my well-being and that I shouldn't hurt their feelings.

I responded by asking, "What about my feelings?"

It had never really dawned on my loving wife that keeping my yard looking nice was something I took great pride in and enjoyed immensely.

I had already mowed the yard several times since the accident, and I knew it was both possible within my new limits and good exercise.

My family had not considered me in their decision, and their actions almost made me feel handicapped – but not quite. After all, I had only lost a leg.

Anger is another major contributor to the new situations that arise, and it can come from any part of the family equation.

Generally speaking, anger starts with the amputee, as he or she blames themself for getting into this situation to begin with, no matter what the reason.

From my experience, men are the worst offenders. Anger at themselves for their condition is fueled easily by family members, who unwittingly say or do things that give the male patient grounds to be even angrier.

The good news is that, if there is love in a household, pity and anger will still show up, but usually find they're not welcome and don't stay very long. That's healthy. It also indicates that the family, as a unit, is on its way to healing and getting on with a life filled with caregiving – not only for the amputee, but for the entire family.

For other families or potential caregiving groups, this welcome scenario never happens – the potential tragedy in every incidence of amputeeism.

You see, when a family member becomes an amputee, every single person in that family is damaged as well.

A huge step towards recovery for the family is dealing with the fact that the amputee is not handicapped!

In my house, I have a saying: **I am not handicapped. I have simply lost a leg.**

You have no idea how much those words helped me to recover.

Obstacles to Overcome

This chapter deals with putting the nuts and bolts of a shattered family back together.

Getting all the family to talk to one another is the hardest part of the healing and bonding process. There is an invisible wall that rises up between an amputee and their family – a wall comprised of many different issues and/or concerns coming from each family member.

Words and actions build the wall, often at a rapid pace, and most of us don't even know construction is underway until the wall is firmly in place.

Components of such walls include these dos and don'ts:

Don't:
- Pity us.
- Be squeamish about the residual limb.
- Discuss us in our absence.
- Assume that a task is automatically something we can't do.
- Over-protect us.
- Make plans that do not include us, while expecting us to be part of them.

Do:
- Encourage us to test our limits.

- Let us determine our own futures as much as possible.
- Remember what we must face daily.
- Help us re-engage with the world.

For a married couple, one of the best steps in shrinking a wall is to formally repeat your wedding vows in front of the entire family. Such an act has a cleansing effect on all involved, allowing the couple to review and reacquaint themselves in their new environment as they now are.

Other family members, who have observed this rekindling of spirit and commitment, often experience far less trouble re-engaging as a family going forward. This can be key to a successful family recovery, because it takes the focus away from the amputee and puts it back on the family, where it should be.

Let's take as an example a family constrained to a one bathroom home. Such a situation requires patience, sharing, scheduling, organization and a multitude of other functions just to keep the house running, even in the best of times.

Families who have overcome the walls erected after an amputation report an honest and workable plan put in place that recaptures the functionality of the family unit, operating under conditions that all know and understand.

Unfortunately, many families never recognize and demolish the walls that have grown up between their members, becoming simply a group of people living under the same roof within a strained environment in a house of glass. Too many times, the glass is broken, and the house comes tumbling down, resulting in destruction of a family.

In the best of all worlds, the limitations of an amputee are seamlessly absorbed into the lives of what should be their most supportive group.

By learning to overcome the issues they now jointly face, a family unit may well find it entirely possible to perform together as a unit even better than before under these new conditions.

Inside an Amputee's Mind

In the period immediately following the amputation of a limb, my own experience tells me that an amputee's mind resembles jelly more than a brain. We are doped to the point where faces of loved ones are distorted, their voices resemble a Saturday morning TV kid's show, and our memories are, for the most part, turned off.

In fairly short order, though, we are returned to some kind of normalcy, and reality begins to emerge.

Pain is the first visitor, and he comes with a vengeance.

At first you are unsure of what has happened to you, because you're really kind of numb all over – the result of the shock your body is experiencing. Then you move a part of yourself where a limb used to be and nothing happens. It is then that Mr. Pain announces his arrival.

Later, with all the people gathered around talking at once in a way that keeps you from understanding much, you feel as if you're in the center ring at a Barnum & Bailey circus.

This, too, fades in a day or so, but now doctors and nurses hover over you, asking all sorts of questions. No matter what comment you make, they all say, "That's good. You're doing just fine. See you in the morning."

Next come the little elf people, who take great delight in sneaking up on you in the middle of the night and waking you up from a perfectly good sleep for one reason or another. I'm sure they have lots of reasons for their actions, but when your brain is on vacation, these reasons don't register.

Of course, the doctors come in the morning, so they can play golf in the afternoon. A nurse must be glued to them, because one is always there so they can be asked to take off the bandage, the doctor wanting to view their masterpiece not touch it!

The doctor asks, "Does that hurt?"

In response, you want to kick him in his manhood and ask him the same question. As luck would have it, he is usually standing on the side of the bed where you have no leg to kick with. I think they practice that.

I can afford a little levity in the above because it is mainly a blur in my mind, even today.

Now things begin to get serious. The professionals demand that you get out of bed and move around.

In my case, I got to see a heavily bandaged stump peeking out from under my gown. Even with my knowledge of what had happened in the wreck, it was a great shock and reality set in hard.

It is in those moments of privacy that you begin to think ahead for the first time. You know what happened by this time and have seen the results, sans prosthesis. It is at this point that thoughts of your future begin to emerge.

Each of us deals uniquely with the possible outcomes. I am blessed with a high degree of determination, and it kicked in early on. Suddenly, I was anxious to get out of bed and even to leave the hospital in order to see what I could make of all this.

I have a strong support group in my family and friends, and for some reason, I did not want to keep them waiting for me. Pushing my doctors and therapy folks, I made good progress despite several additional surgeries.

When my stump and I were allowed to leave the hospital, it was with great expectations on my part, only to have them dashed when I encountered the myriad of obstacles facing me in my own home.

My family had to move all the furniture, so I could get around on the crutches or in my wheelchair. My bedroom is upstairs, but I could not manage the steps, so a hospital bed filled the space where the dining room table used to be. Climbing the stairs became my first goal.

We learn to take our victories in little bites. I have to tell you that mastering the stairs on crutches was huge for me, because it would give me mobility – the first step towards coming back, and I pass that example on to every amputee I talk to as I now have to you.

It was then that a young lady came to call. Her job was to teach me how to stand on one leg without crutches.

Our first lesson began with me standing at the kitchen counter, balancing myself on one leg, and ended with me able to balance myself for fairly long periods of time without holding on to anything – Victory #1!

Several weeks after learning this skill, I was taken to a prosthetics lab to be fitted for my first socket – a very detailed process, including the selection of the type of prosthesis I would use.

Since my amputation was below the knee, I would require an ankle and foot device. Together, the team and I decided on a permanently mounted device that would be attached to the bottom of the socket.

My prosthetists told me there would be several modifications to the socket in the future, as my stump was badly swollen but would reduce itself over time, making the socket too loose to wear as time passed.

During this period, I had to relearn how to stand on two legs, putting more weight on my new prosthesis each time until, finally, I could stand completely upright, although I leaned on a walker for safety's sake.

Holding onto the walker, I took a few steps and was amazed at the fluidity of motion. Those first few attempts weren't pretty, but I was walking – HUGE – Victory #2.

At home, I reviewed the daily maintenance required of my new leg because, to me, that was what my prosthesis was. Such maintenance is a mandatory habit you must develop, if you wish to avoid the list of things that can go wrong and cause you great discomfort, pain and, in some cases, rehospitalization. We'll talk about that in a minute.

As already stated, my first real challenge would be the stairs in my home. How could I navigate them as I now existed?

The walker wouldn't work. That was obvious.

By this time, I was fairly proficient with the crutches, and with my son standing behind me like a backstop, I took the first steps. I was wobbly and shaky, and my son had to catch me several times as I got over-balanced.

I was surprised at how much more difficult I found it to go upstairs fully outfitted with my prosthesis than it had been to go up the stairs with only my remaining leg and my stump. The added weight made a difference.

The next morning, as I was dressing to go downstairs, something wonderful happened. I stood on my own two 'legs' in front of the bathroom mirror and shaved myself - Victory #3!

I walked downstairs that same day, using the stair handrails for balance, and I've been going up and down stairs like that ever since – Victory #4!

Over the next several weeks, I practiced until I could take the steps two at a time in an effort to strengthen my legs, and it worked.

Am I blessed? You bet!

Remember folks, we take our victories, large or small, wherever we find them, and years later, I'm still finding them.

Snapshot – Three

- Caregiving is not taking care of someone. That is care-taking.
- A caregiver does so much more than taking care of someone. Whether short or long term, a true caregiver becomes a part of that person's life in every detail, from the physical things that must be attended to, through the emotional highs and lows, that person travels each and every day.
- While not all forms of caregiving deal with the physical tasks of helping an amputee, they do require in-depth knowledge of that person's physical and mental state.
- A hired caregiver can provide service to the amputee as well as equally important education to spouses and other family members.
- Pity is the worst enemy of an amputee.
- Let the amputee explore his or her limits.
- When a family member becomes an amputee, every single person in that family is damaged as well.
- A huge step towards recovery for the family is dealing with the fact that the amputee is not handicapped!

- In the best of all worlds, the limitations of an amputee are seamlessly absorbed into the lives of what should be their most supportive group.

Maintaining a Prosthesis

Let's talk about maintaining a prosthesis for a bit.

Most come complete with sleeves and liners – two each. They also come with a wide variety of socks to accommodate any short-term changes in the expansion or shrinkage of your stump, which happens daily.

Let me walk you through the maintenance required and how I do mine, just in case you need to know or can learn something new from my experience.

A clean liner is required each day. Roll the liner up from the end of your stump as far as it will go.

Once the liner is in place, slip your stump with its liner into the socket of the prosthesis, checking to see if the device is loose enough to require additional socks, in order to keep a tight fit.

When a good fit has been accomplished, remove the socket and pull a clean sleeve down over it from the top, all the way down to the bottom of the socket – the hard part. Then roll the other loose half of the sleeve down over the socket as well.

Sliding my leg into the socket, I roll the top half of the sleeve up as high as it will go, usually most of the way up my thigh. Making certain there is no slack or bubbles in the sleeve is crucial to keeping the prosthesis held tightly onto the stump and upper leg.

Put weight on the prosthesis to see if the fit is good and tight.

Grabbing an extra sock and a small hand towel, just in case, I'm ready to face the world.

This process will be required to get me ready to walk out the door every morning for the rest of my life.

Compared with wheelchairs, walkers, crutches and the like, the preparations I take each morning are nothing, because the result gives me the mobility and freedom I need to live my life as I want.

The small hand towel and extra sock travel in a back pocket. Depending on various times of the year and amounts of daily exertion, my leg will sweat and the muscles will increase and decrease during a normal day.

If you walk and move around, your muscles will expand, and if you sit at a computer or the like, your muscles will relax and contract some.

Combinations of these movements can make your leg perspire and become slippery. In turn, this allows for some movement of the sleeve down your leg, creating a sag and a loose fit of the socket that soon becomes very uncomfortable and a little dangerous as you move about. Learn to recognize this feeling as you pursue your normal activities. (Remember when mine fell off as I mowed the yard.)

There are two solutions:

A quick fix is simply to roll up your pants, grab the bottom of the sleeve and pull it down until the slack is gone.

Another solution is to feel for the top of your sleeve thru your pants or skirt. Firmly grab hold of the top and your clothing, then pull it up to remove the slack.

Either way works for a temporary fix.

If neither solution solves the problem, find a private spot, pull your clothing down, roll the sleeve down and remove the prosthesis. Take the soft towel, dry both the liner and sleeve completely, and put the prosthesis back. If the socket still feels loose, take it off and add the sock you have with you. Then put it all back on, and you will be good to go.

The final phase every amputee faces is bedtime.

First, go to the bathroom and empty your system for the night.

Second, take your extra sleeve and liner, and wash them in the tub or sink, using a medical soap. Scrub them using your hands. You should use rubbing alcohol instead of soap once a week, and I now use it most times, because it dries quickly and disinfects as well.

Once the sleeve and liner have been rinsed **thoroughly** (otherwise your limb may become extremely irritated the next day from contact with soap residue), hand dry each and hang them from a place near your bed, ready for use the following morning.

Each night when you come in, wash the dirty liner and sleeve you wore that day, allowing them 24 hours to dry before their next use. That way you will always have clean equipment to put on.

If sleeve slippage becomes a problem at any time, take some baby powder and rub it on the top 2-3 inches of the sleeve where it connects with your body. That also works well for me.

Oh, one more thing. I always take a shower, and that poses a problem for a prosthesis since they don't do well in water, especially the new computer driven ones. There are commercial shower legs available for purchase, or you might talk your prosthetists into making you one.

No surprise, I do something different.

I bought a pair of neoprene fishing waders that have soft boot socks instead of regular boots. I cut each to fit above the maximum height of the sleeves I use. Then I conned a nurse out of two, six-inch-wide bands of surgical rubber. They look like giant rubber bands.

Once I have the boot on, I simply roll the surgical rubber to the top of my leg with the prosthetic on and cover the top edge of the fishing boots. It seals the boots tightly against water seepage, and you can walk in and take a shower as if you were on two normal legs.

I keep one shower leg in a travel kit in my truck and another hangs in my shower. I've used this method for four years and have yet to replace any of it.

By the way, I have also gone swimming with my shower leg on, and so far, I've experienced no leaks. Prior to working out this system, I thought about swimming with just one leg and the stump, but knew I'd be swimming in circles.

Another fact of life for an AM (amputee) is return visits to the prosthetic company who built their device. At first, such visits will be frequent, so that the prosthetists can monitor the fit of the prosthesis as the stump changes size.

In my case, the stump swelled considerably as a result of multiple surgeries, and I was told at the start that it would take several months before the swelling would be gone and a better fitting socket could be constructed. In the interim, I had to add or take away layers of socks to maintain a semi-comfortable fit as things settled into place.

To this day, I visit my prosthetics folks at least twice a year and sometimes more often, as sleeves and liners wear out or my stump changes size.

That brings me to the residual limb of any amputation. **Heat and cold, activity and inactivity drive changes in the size of the stump or residual limb.**

For example: If it is a time when outside temperatures have risen, your stump will shrink, mainly due to loss of fluid from perspiration. When active, any muscle increases in size, only to shrink some when inactivity commences. Muscles tend to shrink in cold weather as well.

Any extended swelling or shrinking of the residual limb should be cause for a visit to your prosthetists.

In this chapter, I have tried to show you what an amputee deals with from amputation to finish, day-in and day-out. Hopefully, you now have a better appreciation of the physical, mental, and spiritual strength required of all amputees.

Even those who are still struggling to do everything well deserve our respect and admiration.

Caregiving at Home

This may be the most important part of this book.

You have seen the consuming issues confronting an amputee's daily life. Now let me show you the same issues as they confront the CG (caregiver) in a home life setting.

First things – first. Defining family members and caregiving.

We have briefly discussed caregiving vs caretaking, but it's time for me to help you gain a real understanding of what caregiving means.

A caregiver can best be defined as a care-taker on massive doses of love. Without that one ingredient, the rebirth of a family under these conditions has little, if any, chance of succeeding.

Caregivers must have hearts composed of shoe leather and cotton candy - the size of tomorrow. You see, the strongest caregiver must not only rededicate themselves to the amputee, but to the rest of the family as well, including the CG themselves.

While every member of the family must become a CG, there is always a prime caregiver, and that individual is usually either a mother or a wife. That is simply their instinct.

Hold on a minute, because I have seen many occasions where the dominant female family member is the amputee. What now?

It is always heart-warming and thrilling to me to see a male member of the family step up. It is without doubt the hardest position to fill in this new equation.

Not only must he assume a new role, but he must also learn how to defer to the female amputee's instinctive efforts, so that she can continue in her natural role as much as possible, with total support from him. That's a hard one.

Once they understand this new role, however, many men do a great job of maintaining their positions as heads of households, family planners, along with many other tasks assumed naturally by women. Added to the caregiving role, their plates are mighty full.

Caregiving is a full time commitment that can totally consume a CG. Just like every other vocation in life, we all need a break – time off to refresh our mind and body. Both the CG and AM know that, but in the chaotic state of rebuilding a family unit, it is often forgotten.

Something as simple as a night out, a long lunch or a shopping trip for the lady CGs or, for a man, a few drinks with the his buddies, a fishing trip, bowling tournament or pursuing whatever his hobbies are to name a few can make a huge difference.

You wanna know something else? In planning your timeouts, don't forget the AM. The time away can be just as good for them, because sometimes they need to get away from the family and their CGs, too.

Perhaps we should learn to post signs outside the homes of all new amputees reading:

HOUSE AND FAMILY UNDER RE-CONSTRUCTION

Pardon the humor.

There is much more to follow on this topic, but it is essential that you understand the roles of other members of our families.

Children make up this category for the most part, and in reality, their ages are not too important. What they will learn, understand, and can live are not imaginable to their young minds until they have lived them.

They have seen from birth the images and performances of their parents, and most have built their lives in similar fashion. Now they are faced with radical changes in their perspectives, so how do they deal with them?

The good news is that most children tend to become much closer to each other and the family during such times of trauma, and there is no better word for what has happened in the family life of an amputee than **trauma**.

The youngest children will understand what has happened to Mom or Dad fairly quickly, and their minds tend to make necessary adjustments just as quickly.

Perhaps that is the best age at which to start, as they learn by observation of their siblings and parents. It is logical to assume they will mirror the caregiving shown to them as they grow, and migrate seamlessly into their roles as caregivers in time.

There are countless tales of very young children emulating their parents in doing helpful things. Feeding family pets, helping clear the table, taking out the trash, and even helping the amputee with some personal chore, while the primary CG gets to take a short break. Such children are giving care, and the amputee will return it in kind over time.

These children have no real knowledge of why they are doing these things, but they understand seeing their parents feel better and thrive on the praise coming to them for their efforts. Don't forget the praise part. It's critical.

Teenage to college age family members will be hurt and confused. The rock solid images of both their parents have now been altered, and to convert them into becoming qualified caregivers takes some doing by both the adult caregiver and the amputee – a difficult but necessary endeavor if the family unit is to heal.

Older children's participation is a critical part of the caregiving program in the home. With this group and older, carefully spoken explanations of what the giver and amputee face daily, coupled with eyes on, actual experience of seeing them do their daily routines, allow for great strides in the making of a young caregiver.

For this age group, seeing, understanding and doing are logical progressions. There have been many reports of teens voluntarily modifying their educational and social lives in order to be a more productive part of the caregiving package in the home.

The beauty of that is they make the efforts solely on their own and despite peer pressure from friends, who have no clue what the young person is now dealing with. Not only are these young folks performing critical functions in order to make a potentially dysfunctional family whole again, but they are also being prepared should such an instance happen in their adult lives.

Grown children, living their own lives at different locations than the amputee, are also affected long-term, but the CG-AM syndrome must be viewed differently. After the initial shock of what has happened, grown children pack up their kids and leave for their own homes to live their lives, removed from the new situation.

Loving promises of support are given and, on occasion, actually happen. Often, their solution to the situation is to send money.

While such a gesture can be welcomed and even be critical, it has nothing to do with caregiving. For the most part, however, those distant offspring are so busy that they simply cannot help much. Or can they?

A ten minute phone call can do wonders for both the amputee and caregivers, if it is done in an intuitive, loving way. That is something that must be felt and taught to the callers.

Overtime, both parents, whatever their roles, must teach their adult progeny the right types of calls to make. These must be focused calls, even to specific words, including productive questions, attitude detection, and soft answers to the questions or views being raised from either parent.

Adult offspring can become outside referees and counselors. Who is better equipped?

An Amputee's Homecoming

We have talked briefly about the various roles required of all levels of family caregivers. Let's move on and walk through a homecoming with an amputee and his or her family. Nerves are all on edge, emotions are running strong, and it's not a good time for a mishap, argument or anything that can add to the delicate situation.

Fortunately, there are many things that can be done prior to the homecoming in order to maintain the status quo. There are also some things that should not be done at this point.

Changing material things in the home can cause more issues than any other single factor.

Changes and upgrades must be done in the correct order and manner, if they are to be effective, generally occurring in two phases:

Phase One – Things that a caregiver and the family should do before an amputee comes home to stay.

If you are a spouse or family member, who will be living in the same house with an amputee, you instinctively start thinking about what must be done to accommodate him or her.

A word of caution here: Don't do anything other than the most fundamental and obvious things you think of or see, such as making general access to the house more open, with plenty of room for wheelchairs, walkers or crutches. Clearing paths to bathrooms, bedrooms, primary sitting areas and doorways are but a few of these types of necessary adjustments.

It's okay if you miss some. Phase two details changes you may make during the rest of your lives, and you'll have plenty of time to fix other update requirements as they become obvious, either to you or your amputee.

You may even have to go back and undo some of your preliminary fixes, once you see how your family's amputee reacts. Some folks don't handle change well, even if it means their having to fumble their way around. After all, it is the home they remember, and they are already dealing with a major change.

A good tip is to watch for facial or physical expressions on your amputee's face, when they first get out of the vehicle bringing them home. Let them pause and soak in the view. They have been gone for a while, and they will want to see home as they remembered it in the hospital, longing for things to return to some sort of normalcy.

As they enter the house, let them go as slowly as they want to, and answer every question they ask to their satisfaction.

Once inside, let them choose what they want to do. Don't lead them!

Generally, folks will head for their favorite chair or other piece of furniture. Let them go, only helping if they request or really need it. Tough love? You ain't seen nothing yet!

Bottom line: Making too many changes or offering too much help can unsettle the amputee, establishing them as things you will have to undo or redo.

Your comfort level with your new situation will improve after you have your amputee home and begin to understand what they need and/or want to have done for them.

Phase Two – Things that caregivers and amputees do for each other during the rest of lives together.

So now the amputee is home, and there is a kind of pregnant pause for the entire family, as you all realize how different things really are. Rest assured, this is just the beginning.

At this point, you will learn more about each other as individuals and your family unit than you ever knew or could have imagined, and you don't even get a vote in the matter. Along the way, you will receive several jolts of reality. Be prepared to accept them, because they're surely coming!

Every member of the family has needs that require attention. Solving those needs, back and forth within the family unit, is the essence of caregiving.

No matter what your relationships were before the amputation, even if they were perfect by most standards, they will be radically different now. That is not to say good or bad, just different. Two living beings or more in the case of families will now be required to alter how they live together, if this new situation is to succeed.

Most relationships can muddle through the start of the adjustment process, because all participants will over-extend help to the amputee out of confusion, pity, love, and a myriad of other emotions. At this point, the focus tends to be all about the amputee.

This single-focused viewpoint only works for a short period, then reality sets in.

It is important for you to understand that both sides of the situation actually expect things to return to normal, simply because they can't imagine anything else. Nothing could be further from the truth.

You will find yourselves building anew from the ashes of the old. How you handle that as a family, determines your chances of success or failure!

I have seen 'perfect' families come completely unraveled as their new lives develop, because they can't cope with the changes to their perfect world.

Conversely, some families that were previously hanging on by the thinnest of threads find renewed strength through the changes that are occurring and build on that.

Success or failure hinges on the total family state of mind as the individuals involved approach dealing with the vast numbers of issues now present in their collective lives.

Learning to Give

I have so named this chapter to illustrate that actions and responses must come from all directions and parties involved in daily functions of an amputee household.

Important! - **The relationships between any and all members of an amputee family must be completely candid, totally open, and two-way in order for them to work.**

This means that there must be no inhibitions or hesitations on either side when it comes to dealing with the limb. Yes, I said either side because, at this point in the family's reconstruction, the amputee and caregivers are on the opposite side of the equation until they all learn the meaning of caregiving.

The most delicate aspect of an AM/CG family relationship is that all adjustments stem from a two-sided issue.

For family member CGs, it is completely normal to worry about the things the AM does or tries to do. If your AM tries to do something they did before the amputation, LET THEM TRY. If they succeed, praise them. If they fail, support them – jolt #1.

There is nothing more important than the AM trying desperately to find out what they're capable of now accomplishing, as they restructure their lives. Think about it.

Why would an AM attempt a feat that they are unsure of?

For the most part, it's because they are more concerned about their health and safety than you are. The last thing an amputee wants is to fall down or fumble with something and embarrass either himself or herself and/or their family.

On the other hand, trying to return to a status quo of doing yard work, changing the oil in their vehicles, climbing a ladder or any number of things they have always done is the only path they know to follow.

If you recall, my children hired a yard service for me, when I knew that I could do the work as I always had. I am still not over that.

The absolute wrong things to say to an AM are: *The family is concerned that you might hurt yourself* (doing a thing they had always done, simply because they are now an AM), and/or *If you're injured, you place an increased burden on the family to take care of you.*

How would you like it if, suddenly, for no reason you can fathom, you are denied the freedom to choose what you can and can't do. Sounds like prison to me.

Such constraining comments and/or actions by family CGs will destroy any good they might have intended to do for and/or with the AM, by uttering such uninformed statements as that. This is one of those jolts of reality I mentioned before.

Any AM already feels like they are an increased burden on their family. Now they begin to wonder about their new or perceived lack of quality of life and whether it's even worth living. Rarely do caregivers recognize this condition in an AM – jolt #2.

There are numerous cases where the knowledge of how the family feels, along with the shrinking of things that the AM will be allowed to do, have put AMs in deep depression, accompanied by thoughts as to whether life is even worth living under these conditions. Having experienced these restrictions, I don't blame them.

Family CGs – You have a living breathing family member in your home, who has simply lost a limb. That person is no more a liability to the family unit than they were pre-amputation and certainly no more incapable of living a purposeful and full life than you are. The importance of your avoiding negativity in your relationship with them cannot be overstated.

Regardless of your feelings for the amputee, even if you are someone who feels no more than duty bound to provide care for an AM, family caregivers must allow their AM to reach whatever heights he or she can achieve.

Good, bad, or indifferent, your comments, actions and approaches will inevitably make a difference, positively or negatively in their and the family's lives. Try and put yourself in their shoes. If your roles were reversed, how would you want to be treated?

Believe me, they already have enough on their plates and far more than you do, particularly at this moment, so *Get Over It*!!! Consider this to be another one of those jolts of reality.

Conversely, AMs have a responsibility to the family not to attempt things that are clearly beyond their capabilities.

As a family CG, you must only help when absolutely required and never ignore your AM's need and desire for quality of life, by walking away from your responsibilities as a caregiver.

An amputee fulfilling their true potential will also provide a positive outcome, both for themselves and the caregivers who support them.

Care & Handling of the Prosthesis

As a patient, friend, or caregiver in the hospital, you got to watch as other people handled the residual or stump of the injured limb.

At home, one of the first things an amputee must do is overcome any shyness or reluctance he or she may feel about their handling or letting the appendage be handled. Remember – good, bad, or ugly – what you see is what you are.

The caregiver (CG) can make a real difference by guiding the amputee (AM) into a zone where he or she is comfortable with all family members talking about, looking at, touching and handling that part of the AM, overcoming **all** objections in a warm and loving way.

Upon reaching a workable comfort level, the CG should inspect the limb routinely, looking for anything that may require extra care, and then discuss such needs with the AM. Remember, most AMs can't see the end of their appendage and often don't know if something is awry, until it is raw, painful, or even infected.

Initially, they should jointly wash and clean the stump, using only those materials prescribed by the medical or prosthetics professionals. An infected limb creates a painful situation for the AM, but also deprives them of the thing uppermost to them – the ability to be mobile.

Further, such events create a hardship for the CG in the form of added work to care for the limb.

The care and handling of the modified limb must be an **everyday** activity and can be handled in a number of ways. As life proceeds, most of the care and maintenance will be done by the AM, but the need for a second set of eyes will remain. Remember that!

Inspection and cleaning – by hand:

This can be done by removing any clothing around the stump. Then carefully remove the sleeve, sliding the entire prosthesis off, and then roll off the socks and/or liner. This process will vary some as to the type of amputation, but the general procedure applies to all AMs.

When the AM first comes home, the CG must be careful as the residual limb may still be extremely tender. You will know immediately if that is the case. Adjust your touch accordingly. There may also be stitches or other results of surgery on the limb that may be sensitive as well.

Any raw or open areas should be noted, and that information should be given directly to the medical folks in charge of your case. They will tell you how to proceed. In the meantime, gently wash the entire appendage and pat it dry to avoid tearing any tender skin.

Next, also every day, inspect the portion of the prosthesis sleeve that comes in contact with the AM's skin. Look for rips, holes or abrasions in the device. The best way is to stretch it, while holding it up to a light. Even the smallest of holes will show. You will receive patching instructions from your prosthetists.

A hole in the sleeve or liner means a loss of suction, and the prosthesis will malfunction.

If no rips, holes or abrasions are found, gently wash the sleeve with a very mild soap, using rubbing alcohol only weekly to disinfect. **Bear in mind that water and soap do not do well with the working parts of a prosthesis, so keep them protected as you wash.** Dry with a towel, and stand or lean the device up to allow final drying.

Repeat the above process with the liner.

NOTE: *Many prosthetics companies will provide a rubber, cone-shaped apparatus when shipping a new liner.*

These leftover cones provide the perfect mechanism on which to slide the liner for drying, once it has been put into service. I usually keep two or three of these recycled cones around, so that extra liners can be dried and then stored for the future. It's a good idea to rotate liners daily, so that each will have ample time to dry before use.

The entire prosthesis and all its parts must be kept at bedside for the AM.

Remember the example I used about getting up in the night and falling? That is the absolute last thing that you want to happen, when everyone is in the fledgling stages of learning about the processes that will govern life going forward.

During this initial period, many AMs cannot put their prosthesis on alone, so plan to assist each time, but only as much as the AM needs. They must learn to become independent, and most want to do so as quickly as possible.

Over-assisting will cause friction – guaranteed.

Bathing or showering:

These activities are somewhat complicated at the beginning. Using a tub to sit and soak may be well and good, but getting in and out of a tub can be tricky. Later on, grab bars can be installed, but only when the AM tells you exactly where they want them. The same applies to grab bars around a commode, but that is another story.

Showering is usually the best option, but for most, this should be done as a team effort at first. Let me give you some examples.

Portable shower chairs are available, and they are arguably the best tool for a new AM to use. That said, in the first weeks at home, someone should be in the shower with the amputee or, at least, in position to reach in and assist should the AM become unbalanced or need help bathing.

Money permitting, some families opt to remodel the shower area, by installing a step-in or roll-in shower. Such upgraded facilities usually contain removable shower heads that allow the AM to take a sit-down shower. Included in the package is a fold out chair that can be put up for other family members – a good solution for all.

Note: A fall during any stage of an AM's life will greatly shake the confidence of all concerned, but mostly that of the AM and especially in the first stages of being home.

Standing to shower or hopping about in the early stages of recovery and adaptation are not smart and invariably lead to an accident. Even a plain house stool will provide added stability for the AM and should be provided for their use, if nothing else is available.

As mobility increases, such things as shower legs or boots can be used effectively, allowing the freedom of bathing in privacy.

If there is a downside to using a shower boot, it is that the device remains on in the shower, so the stump must be hand washed afterwards. For me, it is an easy choice, as I prefer to shower alone like any silly, old macho man would. Nevertheless, taking a shower with someone you love, is not all bad!

Snapshot – Four

- A clean liner is required each day.
- A small hand towel and extra sock should travel with an AM all the time.
- If you walk and move around, your muscles will expand, and if you sit at a computer or the like, your muscles will relax and contract some.
- Heat and cold, activity and inactivity drive changes in the size of the stump or residual limb.
- Caregivers must have hearts composed of shoe leather and cotton candy - the size of tomorrow.
- The youngest children will understand what has happened to Mom or Dad fairly quickly, and their minds tend to make necessary adjustments just as quickly.
- Older children's participation is a critical part of the caregiving program in the home.
- A ten minute phone call can do wonders for both the amputee and caregivers, if it is done in an intuitive, loving way.
- Adult offspring can become outside referees and counselors. Who is better equipped?

- Changing material things in the home can cause more issues than any other single factor.
- Changes and upgrades must be done in the correct order and manner, if they are to be effective.
- You may even have to go back and undo some of your preliminary fixes, once you see how your family's amputee reacts.
- Making too many changes or offering too much help can unsettle the amputee, establishing them as things you will have to undo or redo.
- You will receive several jolts of reality. Be prepared to accept them, because they're surely coming!
- Every member of the family has needs that require attention. Solving those needs, back and forth within the family unit, is the essence of caregiving.
- The relationships between any and all members of an amputee family must be completely candid, totally open, and two-way in order for them to work.
- There is nothing more important than the AM trying desperately to find out what they're capable of now accomplishing, as they restructure their lives. Think about it.
- The last thing an amputee wants is to fall down or fumble with something and embarrass either himself or herself and/or their family.
- Conversely, AMs have a responsibility to the family not to attempt things that are clearly beyond their capabilities.
- One of the first things an amputee must do is overcome any shyness or reluctance he or she may

feel about their handling or letting the appendage be handled.

- The CG should inspect the limb routinely, looking for anything that may require extra care, and then discuss such needs with the AM.
- The care and handling of the modified limb must be an everyday activity.
- Every day, inspect the portion of the prosthesis sleeve that comes in contact with the AM's skin.
- A hole in the sleeve or liner means a loss of suction, and the prosthesis will malfunction.
- Water and soap do not do well with the working parts of a prosthesis, so keep them protected as you wash.
- The entire prosthesis and all its parts must be kept at bedside for the AM.
- A fall during any stage of an AM's life will greatly shake the confidence of all concerned, but mostly that of the AM and especially in the first stages of being home.

The Nitty-Gritty of Sharing

Caregiving and receiving in an AM situation is like starting a new marriage with the bonus of previous experience thrown in.

If your marriage before the amputation was filled with love, affection, tenderness and true feelings for each other, you are blessed. If not, you have an opportunity to restart all that by sharing the new situation with each other.

The key to success is simple: Pay attention to each other! **Pay attention to each other! Pay attention to each other!**

Even in the best of relationships, we tend to think of ourselves first. That is old school, outdated, and selfish, and yes, I have a strong opinion.

In order for this new situation to grow and mature successfully, both parties, indeed all of those involved, must train themselves to think of themselves, their partners, and others in the relationship – all at the same time.

"Let's see. I need to go to the store." And then, "Does it affect my partner in any way?"

Just finished taking a shower. Did I leave it in condition for anyone with or without special needs to use it?

Just finished running the vacuum. Did I return it to the closet?

Have I picked up dirty clothes, and put them in the hamper, instead of piling them on the floor?

I dropped those folded clothes on the steps, so I can take them up later. Will they be in the way?

Moved the footstool from in front of the couch, so I could have room for my prosthesis. Did I put the stool back for others to use?

Just changed and cleaned liners for my prosthesis. Did I put everything back where they belong?

Is the thing I plan to do going to upset my family?

The list is endless, and the solution is a hard habit to master. If you look carefully, many of the things I cited above, are the same things we deal with in a non-AM family. Stop a moment, and remember how many arguments they have caused.

Multiply that by the intensity of every AM family, and at the very least, you have a recipe for discord. Every single thing you do, whether amputee or caregiver, has a direct or future impact on the other.

Until you adopt that mindset, your household is at risk of tragedy. Keep in mind that psychologists tell us it takes three weeks of repetition to develop a habit, a cautionary reminder for those experiencing the initial three weeks at home with a new amputee.

You will see me refer to this type of mental process throughout the book. In truth, I can't say it enough.

Even after years of working in a loving, amputee household, both my wife and I have mental lapses and forget. Fortunately, we both understand that even with the right habits built, we are human. It is then that the strength of our relationship kicks in, and we forgive.

Without that capacity, you are walking down a slippery slope, from which many do not recover.

While many pitfalls exist in such a relationship, it really isn't that different from a 'normal' family's requirements for healthy and safe living. The difference is the intensity with which you must monitor your actions as you strive to live safely and happily together.

The caregiver has had to face the reality that the spouse is not the same person as before, and the amputee must recognize that the entire family has made major lifestyle changes on his or her behalf.

These changes result in two things:

1. The highs are much higher when they occur, and
2. The lows are terrible – filled with hurt, anger and even fear.

Let me explain. When something really good happens between an AM and their CG, the emotions running through both of them are escalated higher than the norm, because they have traveled together along a path rarely experienced by others.

When lives have been at risk, as in an AM situation, all senses are heightened by the possibility of further loss. Emotions associated with such events become permanent residents in the minds of those involved and remain close to the surface.

By contrast, the family who has never been exposed to such a situation hasn't felt anxiety, fear and worry to this degree. Because most family members have never come close to losing a spouse, parent, child, or sibling, they've never experienced such feelings. They can't even imagine the death of a loved one, because they don't wish to deal with it and simply put it aside.

Another issue in the realm of nitty-gritty is the fact that an AM will have some continuing pain or discomfort for the rest of their life. So, no matter how well they walk and get around, there will be times when they are hurting.

The CG must learn to look for the signs, because often the AM will have become resigned to the pain, but that doesn't mean they aren't in distress and need assistance, especially if the pain is generated by irritation or, even worse, infection.

Phantom Pain – Real or Myth?

I believe the general consensus believes that what an amputee feels mimics felt pain, but in actuality it is only in the mind of the AM. I can tell you the first time it hit me as I lay in my hospital bed, a couple of days after my wreck, I didn't care where it came from, it just hurt like blazes.

It began as a series of tingling sensations from my non-existent leg, so real that I actually looked under the sheet to see if it was there. That's the truth. The feelings were so familiar and comfortable, that they over-rode my actual knowledge of the loss.

That feeling quickly gave way to a jolt of intense pain that stayed with me for about an hour. Confused, I pressed the button, and a young nurse walked in. When she saw I was in pain, she immediately sent for the doctor. The chief of the surgical team who had worked on me came in shortly after the pain subsided and educated me, using a computer for his example.

Using the computer – brain analogy, he pointed out that my brain had experienced a major crash with subsequent residual damage, similar to those we're accustomed to hearing about with computers.

During the process of rebooting, such a computer tries to reach software that has been destroyed in the crash, working to reconnect with open softwares, until it finally gives up and leaves a message on the screen telling the user of its findings.

These computers will continue to open the other programs as normal. However, they will send similar error messages each time they are restarted, until the destroyed software is replaced or deleted.

Recovering from a similar 'crash,' my brain had awakened from the surgery and attempted to reconnect with all my body parts. When it reached the place where my leg had been, it tried to contact parts of the leg that no longer existed, using thousands of electronic messages.

Failed communications with the missing limb and responding messages from adjoining nerves then sent signals back to my brain telling it that something was wrong, thereby creating the tingling sensations I felt.

Those signals appeared to have come from the area where my leg used to be. While the computer could pop a window on its screen to send that message, my brain did what it could do and sent pain as its way of telling me something was wrong. Now I understood completely.

Phantom tingling and pain is real, as any amputee will tell you. In some cases, it doesn't begin for several weeks or months, and in others, like mine, it came in a hurry.

How long will such pain last?

Mine usually hung around for thirty minutes to an hour and visited me daily for about a week. For others, the time of duration is much longer and can go on, intermittently, for months.

Some folks have much later occurrences. I have brief, but infrequent, periods of phantom pain years after my accident took place in 2006.

My solution to making the pain go away is purely mental. I *will* it away.

Now I know that sounds unlikely, but I simply get angry, focusing that anger on the pain and my mind on the real knowledge that the leg is no longer there, until my brain gives up and the pain goes away. I can only tell you that it works for me.

Phantom pain is one of the things I alluded to earlier that will cause an AM to experience periods of pain in their lives, and therefore, it's another of the things CGs must be aware of, as they care for an AM.

Beyond the Shower

I hinted that we might discuss commodes earlier, and while it can be a crappy topic, it bears flushing out.

Most homes have the original commode that came with it. For all amputees, the device needs to be the sixteen inch tall model, often referred to as comfort height, to make it easier for them to stand and sit down, minimizing balance issues and helping to prevent falls.

It is relatively easy to switch an old commode for a new one, and some of the newest models can even be flushed by simply waving a hand over them. In cases of an AM who has lost an arm, it's a good idea to get a toilet paper dispenser mounted on a stand that can be moved to accommodate them.

In addition to a taller commode, grab bars on both sides provide valuable assistance for both sitting and standing. Such bars are easily found in many department, box, and home improvement stores. The key to installation is to make certain that they are firmly bolted into the floor or wall studs strong enough to bear the weight of the AM.

Throw rugs are commonly used in bathrooms, especially those with tile floors. At a minimum, such rugs must have thick rubber backing to prevent slippage. An AM coming out of a shower or getting up from the commode, depends heavily on a firm surface to take those first few steps.

I remind you that a fall damages an AM's self-confidence, but it also undermines the confidence of the

AM's family as to their competence to cope independently with daily routines, even though the fall may not have been the fault of the AM.

As amputees, we have tendencies to revert to how we moved around pre-amputation, simply because we have more information stored in our brains from past experiences, than we do new information that we are gathering about our current mobility requirements. Old habits are hard to break.

Arguments over issues pertaining to the AM's handicap are no-win scenarios for everyone concerned.

During such arguments, old aggravations, such as leaving the toilet seat up or down, not replacing the toilet paper roll, missing the toilet with an errant squirt or two and the like are often drawn into the discussion, further muddying the water. Some things never change!

Reviewing the rest of the bathroom, there are some other things to note. One such concern is a hard area for our ladies.

We guys know that you gals love to have all your feel good, smell even better, and look wonderful goodies about you on the counter in the bath. Most of us fellows will agree that equality in the bathroom has long been a myth.

You gals might consider, though, that an AM – yes, even a man – will now require items to be left there, too, simply to avoid the balancing and juggling involved just get dental, smell good and shaving equipment from under the counter.

Here's a picture:

Joe finishes his shower and either needs a place in the shower or in the bathroom, where he can reattach his prosthesis. He should not have to hop or use crutches to reach a seat.

Once the prosthesis is mounted, be it an arm or a leg, there is the issue of getting to the sink where he will continue his ablutions. If it's an arm, then walking is not too much of an issue, except that if Joe slips, he now has but one limb with which to catch himself. On the other hand, said facetiously, if his is a leg amputation, several points should be considered.

First, he will not have on the shoes that normally stabilize his walking. Next, even with a sock on over his foot, bathroom floors can be slippery and, therefore, present a serious hazard, especially if he must deal with stepping back and forth from a tile floor to a small throw rug or rugs. What Joe needs is a path close to objects that he can grab or hold onto as he navigates his way.

Finally, the CG should **NEVER** leave things, such as a pile of dirty clothes, anywhere on the floor of the bathroom. **Such items are a recipe for disaster.**

Here's why. In nearly all cases, a leg AM fails to develop early feelings for just how long their prosthesis is. You see, their brain now senses only to the end of the stump, leaving the prosthesis no more than a stick hanging from the stump. This means that an AM has no sense of height as they step over an object.

During the initial days after my accident, I must have tripped over a mile of objects – not because I failed to see them, but because my brain couldn't calibrate how high I would have to lift my leg, with its attached prosthesis, to step over them.

Time is a great healer of that shortfall, as AMs eventually learn to over compensate the height of things in their way, but in the beginning it is a real issue for us.

Closets are another thing that is often found in the general vicinity of the bathroom. Easy moving or no doors at all on closets placed in this area provide a good solution for the AM.

Once inside a closet, extra lighting will be required to insure that our Joe can easily maneuver through his shoes, boots, extra prosthetic accessories, and the wall of clothing hanging in front of him.

It wouldn't hurt to ask Joe where he would like to have a grab-bar or two mounted for his convenience. He probably won't think to ask for it.

Now we have spent quite a bit of time here in the bathroom, but it is the one place where I felt I could show you the best examples of ideas that help CGs and AMs alike to tread successfully, without creating the basis for arguments. That has happened before, hasn't it?

My spouse and I still have disagreements, but we promised that they would never be about my issues. Instead, things like who stole the toothpaste, left fingerprints on the mirror, unplugged her hair-curler, or spilled powder all over the counter occupy our time.

Arguments between AMs and CGs are never productive. Both should go somewhere, cool off, and then approach the issue again.

There is no argument that can't be solved, as long as there is love involved.

Adapting

In previous chapters, we have discussed the need for complete candidness when dealing with an amputated limb. Let's talk about an area which often becomes a huge stumbling block in AM/CG relationships – SEX!

Oh, so you haven't thought about that one yet, huh? Okay, let's talk about it now.

The need and desire for sex generally remains after an amputation, but can be clouded in a host of issues that can wreck a sexual relationship, if they aren't dealt with early on.

Earlier, we discussed the need to openly confront the look, touch and feel of an amputated limb by the CG. The most important aspect of this is to make certain that both the AM and the CG accept and become used to these. This can take time and a lot of patience.

Let's assume for a minute, that both of you have gotten past all that and are dealing successfully with the issues of daily living. Suddenly one or the other is struck by the primal urge in all of us for sex, as can happen in a myriad of ways. Looking, touching, feeling by chance are but a few of the triggers.

For the AM, there many possible complications that immediately fill their mind. Can I perform? Will my partner be able to deal with how I perform?

Then comes the biggie. I can't do it the normal way. How do we deal with that?

In the case of breast removal or implantation, a woman will often be concerned with how she now looks to her partner. Will the sight of her naked body still arouse him?

CGs also have issues. This is the person I married and love, but how can we do this without causing pain or embarrassment? What if I hurt my mate? Will it damage our sex life or, even worse, our relationship if, the first time we try, things don't go well?

You know what? The above are all valid issues, and there are many more.

Here's one that must be mentioned - For ladies, it is huge - Handling the mastectomy mentality.

You have heard me say and will continue to hear that the only place AMs are handicapped is between their ears. While that is true, there are a couple of new players in the lives of mastectomy amputees: Mystique and Allure.

Most men do not have a clue about what that means to a woman, but all you ladies do. Breasts or the lack of them are critical from your perspective.

There are a growing number of women whose self-confidence is well established. They exude an attitude of take me like I am or not at all. Hopefully, that mindset would be of great value to a mastectomy amputee, but what about the rest of you?

Are you the same woman you were? Of course, you are. You are simply missing a breast or two. It cannot affect your inner being unless you let it!

You are still the wonderful person you have always been, and that is what men see more than anything else (believe it or not). Add to that the amazing new procedures available that return you to the same basic symmetry you had before, and with your clothes on, who knows?

How do you deal with the dreaded explanations? The same way the rest of us amputees do, with truthful and candid responses.

For those who have a personal need to know –
husbands, lovers, the curious child, and others you deem
necessary, bare all to the world. Let them touch, feel and
ask all the questions they want. The process takes away
their concerns, but more importantly, your concerns about
acceptance are answered first hand by those closest to you.

Once you have dealt with the nitty-gritty of your
situation, finding that those who you need to love and adore
you still do, then you can return to fulfilling the feminine
mystique and allure you thought missing. You will find that
it never left.

I won't pretend to know the solutions to all of the issues
re sex, but one thing I do know. There is not a single issue
regarding sex that can't be solved, as long as you were
enjoying normal sex before the amputation.

You know something else? I've been told that a post-
amputation sex life can be great, even if sex between the
partners prior to the amputation wasn't all that good. That's
right.

When all the emotional buttons have been pushed
leading up to that moment of intimacy, many partners don't
really notice the obvious changes, as they are too focused
in love-making. In the post-physical part of making love,
many couples have found great tenderness and even some
humor in the adaptations they made 'on the fly' as it were.

For example, a woman with an arm AM found that she
used her remaining limb and increased movement in her
lower body and face to offset what could have been a
shortfall. A man with the same issue, found that changing
positions made the difference for he and his partner. A
paraplegic man found that being on the bottom of the
coupling worked well and actually improved his climax.

The adaptations above are but a few of the many
creatively successful ways for AMs and CGs to make
warm, wonderful love and enjoy intensely satisfying sex.

Key to all of this is openness, willingness to try changes, and the ability to laugh about any experiments that don't work. After all, it's a new world to both partners, although it can be exciting and rewarding.

For those couples whose lives are based on loving one another and adhering to the wedding vows 'for better or worse,' post amputation sex is simply another way for them to grow closer.

Far and away, the most important organ to use well, when seeking a successful love life is your mouth!

TALK ABOUT WHAT WILL MEET THE NEEDS OF AND SATISFY BOTH OF YOU AS MUCH AND AS MANY TIMES AS IT TAKES.

If you can't bring sex into the open with words of understanding and verbal descriptions of what can make it better, it will never be better, if it exists at all.

Keeping up Appearances

By this time, you all know about my amputated BK leg, and while this chapter title would appear to be facetious to some, it isn't.

Let me explain. Before I was able to get into a prosthesis, I felt it necessary to go back to work. I gathered up my crutches, folded my pant leg over the stump or residual limb, pinned it up, and out the door I went.

My first stop was to the home of an elderly lady who had met me before the accident. When I walked in her door, she cried, tried to hug my neck, and became so distracted that I finally told her, I would be back later. I wasn't the same to her, and she didn't handle it well. Lesson learned.

The next day, I made a first time visit to a couple, who spent so much time looking at where my lower leg had been and making consoling statements, that I again excused myself with a promise to return soon.

The following day was spent with a prosthetist getting fitted. I was gonna solve that problem once and for all.

One month later, I revisited the first lady mentioned above. She was delighted to see me with two 'good' legs, my roper boots, cowboy hat and a minor limp. We did not discuss the leg.

The couple I had visited was a little reluctant on the phone, but to give them credit, they agreed to a second meeting. Walking into their home, I was a revelation to them. They kept asking how I was managing to do so well and stating that I didn't look at all like I was crippled.

By the time I left, I believe they understood when I said, "I'm not crippled or handicapped. I have simply lost a leg." Then I added, "If you see it around here anywhere, please call and let me know."

You know the old comedic saying, "Keep 'em laughing!"

Summers in Texas can get a mite hot. As with anybody, else, Bermuda shorts came in handy, but for me they came with a price.

By now, I had a prosthesis – bare metal and a rubber foot. When I wore shorts, folks could see all that ugly metal device starting below the socket and sleeve. Because my prosthesis looked nothing like a normal leg, folks had a hard time dealing with it. On the other hand, kids were totally in awe of it, wanting to touch and feel it as they asked a million questions.

So...

Back to the prosthetists, I went. They measured my other leg, and I came away with some flesh-colored wrapping that completely hid the metal device and matched my whole leg exactly. While it does add some weight to my leg, it has been immensely successful for me.

There was one catch I discovered after I had worn a wrapped prostheses in summer with shorts. When my natural leg began to tan, my lovely wife threatened to put make-up on the prosthesis, so it would match.

Out in the world, most people simply want to know how I hurt my knee. A wrapped device is a great solution for anyone who is a BK AM.

The other thing that really helped me to keep up appearances – practice walking until you limp so slightly that folks don't know what's going on under your trouser leg(s), dress, or even when you're wearing shorts.

All I can say here is practice, practice and practice some more. Use a mirror, and request critiques from those around you, until even they can't see a limp.

Is this being a narcissist? No. It is simply you as an AM paying it forward to those around you, by showing that you care enough about them to look your best. Of course, it won't hurt your ego either.

In the case of those you might be honored to counsel, your own appearance could be the boost they need to get them up and moving towards their own recoveries. Eventually, they, too, may have a chance to counsel others, and that keeps the circle going, doesn't it?

Snapshot – Five

- **The key to success is simple:** Pay attention to each other! **Pay attention to each other! Pay attention to each other!**
- The caregiver has had to face the reality that the spouse is not the same person as before, and the amputee must recognize that the entire family has made major lifestyle changes on his or her behalf.
- When lives have been at risk, as in an AM situation, all senses are heightened by the possibility of further loss.
- Another issue in the realm of nitty-gritty is the fact that an AM will have some continuing pain or discomfort for the rest of their life.
- The CG must learn to look for the signs, because often the AM will have become resigned to the pain, but that doesn't mean they aren't in distress and need assistance, especially if the pain is generated by irritation or, even worse, infection.
- The general consensus believes that what an amputee feels mimics felt pain, but in actuality it is only in the mind of the AM.

- Phantom tingling and pain is real, as any amputee will tell you. In some cases, it doesn't begin for several weeks or months, and in others, like mine, it came in a hurry.
- My solution to making the pain go away is purely mental. I will it away.
- Arguments over issues pertaining to the AM's handicap are no-win scenarios for everyone concerned.
- In nearly all cases, a leg AM fails to develop early feelings for just how long their prosthesis is.
- There is not a single issue regarding sex that can't be solved, as long as you were enjoying normal sex before the amputation.
- Post-amputation sex life can be great, even if sex between the partners prior to the amputation wasn't all that good.
- Far and away, the most important organ to use well, when seeking a successful love life is your mouth!
- A flesh-colored wrapping around the prosthetic is a great solution for anyone who is a BK AM.
- The other thing that really helped me to keep up appearances – practice walking until you limp so slightly that folks don't know what's going on under your trouser leg(s), dress, or even when you're wearing shorts.
- In the case of those you might be honored to counsel, your own appearance could be the boost they need to get them up and moving towards their own recoveries.

The Test of Time

I'm sure that, over time, most AMs and their CGs settle into a pattern of living. As an AM, I fight this every day.

Why? Because with a pattern of living comes complacency and settling for what you are – a fairly common occurrence among us, due primarily to the extras that we deal with in daily life. Often, we get caught up where we are, as opposed to where we could be.

Never do that.

Force yourself to start every day looking for some way to improve yourself, not just relying on the normal processes you use to get up and get going. Extend this to include getting a better job, more education, and a better status in life. At the same time, stay alert for any changes in the medical world or new equipment that can enhance or even replace the prosthesis you now have.

Push yourself to do more at home, to get more deeply engaged in what all the CGs around you are doing. That is how you pay back, in part, for all the care they have shown you.

The bottom line here is: keep occupied all the time.

The goal is for you to look down to where you started as an AM and up to where you are now. Keeping your eye on this ball will make your life much more meaningful to you and to those around you.

Improvements in the medical world dealing with amputees, amputations, and the equipment amputees use are improving mobility for all of us. Just think, computer driven hands, arms and legs are but a few of the things changing almost daily. The latest thing I saw was a hand actually tied to the nerves in a man's brain that allowed the user's brain to tell his hand what to do.

In my own case, my foot is now computerized, telling the prosthetic foot when to bend and how much to do so as I walk. This computer allows for near normal heel and toe movement, which makes a big difference, believe me.

My computerized device also controls the angle of my ankle. If I walk across a slanted surface, it automatically corrects my leg to the proper vertical position. Wonderful news to an AM, right?

I'm looking forward to the day when my brain can tell both of my feet to dance a jitterbug with my lovely wife. I dream of doing things I must think of step by step now just by relying on normal movement.

Pursue anything new, as if you were a man in the desert who, dying of thirst, sought an oasis. Also seek out programs that can fund such things for you, in case your insurance doesn't.

Hard to find? Yes, but what a small price to pay to get you closer to the normal that you once had.

Let your family and other CGs know what you are seeking. They can be of great help through their use of television, computer searches, and social media. Remember this, nearly all of the latest trends in medical news appear first on Twitter and/or Facebook, as well as through other social media, long before traditional media gets it.

I receive messages from family members almost daily, pointing out something new.

"Hey, Dad, did you see the story about this or that?" What they send may not be what you're looking for, but the joy of knowing that family and friends care enough to be in the hunt with you is priceless.

It stimulates me to forward that information to other AMs I know, and that type of action helps keep the circle of AMs alive and well. Everyone pays it forward.

Speaking of paying it forward, there are a wide variety of support groups, usually made up of amputees who are openly willing to discuss their issues in order to help other AMs, who are in trouble at home or at work.

These selfless folks pay it forward in ways most of you can't begin to understand. Imagine an AA meeting where everyone exposes themselves mentally, except that here it is both mental and physical exposure.

If you find yourself, as a CG or AM, unable to cope with your situation at home, such support groups can provide valuable advice and assistance from folks who can both walk the walk and talk the talk. Never hesitate to find help wherever it may be. Maybe one day, you too can pay it forward.

Any prosthetist and many AMs/CGs will know where the nearest group meets.

Back to the nitty-gritty. **Over time, expect changes in your residual limb.**

Even if you remain active and keep the muscles developed, there will be a certain amount of shrinkage. You know the drill. More socks and, eventually, a new socket will accommodate the shrinkage. This is as normal a part of the aging process as losing your hair, so don't panic.

If you go from a period of inactivity to being active, expect to take off socks as needed to allow the socket to fit properly. Remember, we AMs are carrying at least one extra sock in our hip pocket or purse.

You may also experience increases in pain, particularly if you over-exercise.

These episodes are no different from what happens when we use any other muscle that we have stopped using as we age. It just feels like it hurts more than before. This pain, too, will go away with more exercise, some liniment and, who knows, perhaps a shot of "Who Hit John?"

If you are a young AM, your normal activity rate may preclude the above mentioned side issues from happening. If such discomfort does arise, though, contact your prosthetics company or your orthopedic surgeon. It might be something else.

As Time Goes By

You are about to embark on a doom and gloom episode, so sit deeper in your chair and open your sensibilities.

Our natural bodies go through a host of changes as we age. We all know that, and it just aggravates the daylights out of us. For some AMs, a different scenario crops up.

Since few of us age gracefully, we tend to grumble and moan about our physical equipment wearing down and the fact that it often must be augmented by synthetic devices like glasses, contacts, shoe supports, canes, walkers, braces, countless pills, and a host of other things.

There is a very subtle change occurring in each of us as that happens, and it goes back to something I spoke about in the front of this book. I called it TATLOH – Two Arms, Two Legs, and One Head – equal and not separate. The example I used described a natural situation among young children and their peer groups.

TATLOH applies in a different way for aging. Most of us got past that discriminatory stage as we matured into adults, going about our lives in as normal a condition as we could and blending into the social background like everybody else.

With the introduction of synthetic devices into our lives, many folks experience a subtle but impactful change in their own attitudes. No longer do they fit the adult version of TATLOH. Now, in some almost unrecognizable way, things are no longer the same.

In a different, yet similar way, we return to that youngster going to school for the first time as we, once again, face the social acceptability issues of our childhoods. The difference is sometimes hard to see in the aging process.

If you don't believe that and are not handicapped, borrow a walker from someone and spend one day using it as a normal part of your moving about. Not only will you experience the hardships of dealing with the device, but if you don't experience the change in attitudes towards you by your peers and many others you come in contact with, I'll kiss your foot.

The change will be hard to see at first. It ranges from looks of pity and concern, to diminishing eye contact and even avoidance.

Aging is a process of returning to non-acceptance by our peers, similar to what we experienced when we were kids.

Unfortunately, it seems to be a product of our society, where the respect previously held for elders has gone away, replaced by 'Sorry. You are no longer one of us.' The impact on those of us in that situation can easily be seen.

The next time you're out in public, make a special effort to locate and observe folks using a walker or wheelchair. They're easy to find. Heads down, making no eye contact, and nearly always appearing apologetic for their conditions, they go about their lives.

There's another group of people using devices, and you will see them as well, if you look. These are the folks who are angry because they must use an aid of some type and are even angrier at the treatment they are given by their former peers. You can find them at bus stops, in checkout lines at your local store, and in most public places. Imagine the difficulty facing those folks.

I used the above to illustrate that nearly all of us, AMs or not, are headed in that direction by virtue of the fact that we all get old.

There is another interesting observation that can be gleaned from your observance of older people. Watch to see how they are treated by members of our society who are AMs. I've often witnessed what appears to be a kind of bonding, apparently formed out of commonality and shared experience.

What can be learned from the above material you just read?

While not always a hardship, being different is always difficult. Being different, by exhibiting a physical impairment of any kind, is life changing at any age.

What Have We Learned?

I can't speak for you readers, but as the author, I learned a great deal.

Losing a limb, means exactly and only that.

You have lost a limb. Whether you become handicapped by that loss is up to you as an amputee and your caregivers. Such a loss should never become a handicap.

Remember this: Amputees learn to take our victories in little bites.

Whether a child or senior, anyone with a handicap, I detest that word, must enter a new lifestyle after the event occurs that places them in that position. Some adapt and make it just fine. Others don't and fall by the wayside.

We know that there is a significant difference between caretakers and caregivers. The latter are separated into two groups: those who care for their patients (AMs) long term and are paid for service and those who are family members, ranging from spouses to children and, occasionally, others in the family unit.

Amputees and caregivers must develop a symbiotic relationship, with each contributing to the other's needs, in order for the overall relationship to return as close to normal as possible or even to be enriched.

AMs face formidable adaptations to their lifestyles, and without caregivers, many simply can't make life work. The greatest tool for creating a workable relationship is simple and, at the same time, difficult – **PAY ATTENTION TO EACH OTHER!!!**

Place no limits on the amount of caregiving between the CG and the AM. Notice the AM must return care evenly.

AMs and CGs alike must recognize and learn to deal with the additional tasks facing the AMs, daily for the remainder of their lives.

Once a CG, always a CG. CGs must know as much or more than the amputee about the care and maintenance of his or her prosthesis.

Phantom pain is real to the amputee.

Both must create or rekindle the type of relationship that enhances each, in order for them to live and grow together.

Renewing an AM/CG's couple's wedding vows is a good way to refresh emotions that have possibly dimmed over time. Done in front of family members, it can draw the family closer as a unit, thereby making the CG/AM transition smoother.

Amputees should and, generally, do push the envelope of their new capabilities, and all CGs in the family must encourage, not discourage, their efforts. Allowing an AM to learn about themselves and grow with this new knowledge is crucial. AMs must never become complacent or fall into the realm of the status quo, and CGs must ensure these bad habits don't develop.

Never say or do anything about the amputee without their participation and permission.

Most important, never let an AM see, hear or feel that they are a burden to the rest of the family. If you do, any efforts and progress made will be lost, and you may lose the AM as well.

All parties must keep aware of any improvements in the equipment required by the AM, and such improvements should be discussed with the AM as to possible benefits.

AMs – look your best. When you look good, you feel good, and those around you will feel so as well. CG/family - when your AM looks good –TELL THEM!!

A note for folks in general: Why not pass out a little praise and admiration for the person whose life has been unalterably changed? Example: "Don't stare like that, honey. Just think what a wonderful person he/she must be. Living with a missing limb must really be hard."

A wise man once said, "It takes a war to awaken the medical community as to the needs of all those who suffer."

I salute all our young men and women who woke the medical community, at such great damage to thousands, to get us where we are today in supporting the processes involved in dealing with an amputation and the development of the prosthetic tools now available.

A rule for all amputees - ***Think through it, before you do it.*** Works every time.

Finally, all amputees, caregivers and every other soul on the planet is headed towards a time when prosthetic or other aid devices are required. *IT'S CALLED AGING.*

As you make your journey in life, remember that, at some point, others will see you as they see amputees. Unless you wish to be treated the way they are, change how you feel now. It will affect all those around you and who knows how many others.

My thoughts are with every person who is an amputee, a caregiver or in some way capable of affecting one of their lives.

I wrote this because of them and those who will inevitably follow or, in a word, everyone.

D. A Grady

Amputee

D. A. Grady

D.A. Grady has spent much of his life in the west. Growing up, high school summers were spent chasing mustangs or wild horses, just outside of Reno, Nevada, where he and friends captured and broke them to ride, later selling them for school money.

A veteran, old school cowboy, he is most at home in that world, including, hunting, fishing and spending time with his animals.

After joining the U.S. Navy in 1962, he received a Presidential appointment to the Naval Academy, after which he rejoined the fleet and became part of America's space program. While stationed aboard the USS Lake Champlain, he worked in air traffic control and was a member of the team used to recover Gemini III and Gemini V space vehicles.

Later, he joined the news staff of KSWO-TV in Lawton, Oklahoma, where he anchored the news desk for several years, during which he received the Salvation Army's National Service to Mankind Award for a documentary he produced on nearby Snyder, Oklahoma, after it was devastated by a tornado.

In years to follow, D.A. entered U.S. Army civil service at Ft. Sill, Oklahoma, as a logistician working in emergency management, designing and operating a first of its kind emergency operations center that played a key role in Operation Desert Storm.

During that time, he undertook the training of specialized dogs used in the detection of narcotics and explosives. He and his dog, King, were known nationwide for their efforts in detecting contraband in both military and federal law enforcement.

Later, he transferred to Ft. McPherson, Georgia, to become the Chief of the Army's Away Team – a rapid response deployment unit, providing on-site management and reporting to the highest levels of the Pentagon.

Recruited by Dell Computer, D.A. came to Austin, Texas, where he worked as operations manager for its federal division.

Two years later he formed Solutions for Older Americans, LLC, a consulting firm, working exclusively with America's senior citizens in an effort to help them improve their quality of life.

Mr. Grady lives in Cedar Park, Texas, with his wife, Emma. His sons, Ken and Carl, live in Houston and daughter Angela lives close by.

He can be found at his website: www.bardsnest.com and also at his blogsite: http://wp.me/p5Bnng-qS.

You may follow him on Twitter as @dagsnotes.

www.ingramcontent.com/pod-product-compliance
Lightning Source LLC
Chambersburg PA
CBHW072210280526